SUPER
SEARCHERS
on HEALTH
& MEDICINE

**The Online Secrets of Top
HEALTH AND MEDICAL RESEARCHERS**

SUPER
SEARCHERS
on HEALTH
& MEDICINE

The Online Secrets of Top
HEALTH AND MEDICAL RESEARCHERS

Susan M. Detwiler
Edited by Reva Basch

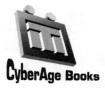

CyberAge Books

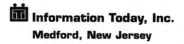
Information Today, Inc.
Medford, New Jersey

First Printing, 2000

Super Searchers on Health and Medicine:
The Online Secrets of Top Health and Medical Researchers

Super Searchers, Volume IV
A series edited by Reva Basch

Liability

Trademarks

Library of Congress Cataloging-in-Publication Data
Detwiler, Susan M., 1953-
　　Super searchers on health & medicine : the online secrets of top health and medical researchers / Susan M. Detwiler ; edited by Reva Basch.
　　　　p.cm. – (Super searchers ; v. 4)
　　Includes bibliographical references and index.
　　ISBN 0-910965-44-7
　　　　1. Medicine—Computer network resources. 2. Medicine—Information services. 3. Internet (Computer network) 4. Medical informatics. I. Title: Super searchers on health and medicine. II. Basch, Reva. III. Title. IV. Series.

R119.9 .D486 2000
025.06'61—dc21　　　　　　　　　　　　　　　　00-043006

Printed and bound in the United States of America

Publisher: Thomas H. Hogan, Sr.
Editor-in-Chief: John B. Bryans
Managing Editor: Janet M. Spavlik
Copy Editor: Dorothy Pike
Production Manager: M. Heide Dengler
Cover Designer: Jacqueline Walter
Book Designer: Jeremy M. Pellegrin
Indexer: Laurie Andriot

Dedication

To my mother, Anna Pallas, of blessed memory, who told me,
"How do you know, if you don't try?"

About The Super Searchers Web Page

At the Information Today Web site, you will find *The Super Searchers Web Page*, featuring links to sites mentioned in this book. We will periodically update the page, removing dead links and adding additional sites that may be useful to readers.

The Super Searchers Web Page is being made available as a bonus to readers of *Super Searchers on Health and Medicine* and other books in the Super Searchers series. To access the page, an Internet connection and Web browser are required. Go to:

www.infotoday.com/supersearchers

Table of Contents

Foreword

by Stephen Barrett, M.D.

Access to medical information is growing at an amazing rate. Information experts are key participants in this process. *Super Searchers on Health and Medicine* consists of ten interviews with medical librarians, independent researchers, and others who use their training to find evidence-based information for medical professionals, consumers, and anyone else who needs it. It discusses sources, search techniques, and career pathways. It's a quick, easy read, filled with nuggets of personal experience.

Desktop computers now provide doctors and patients with ready access to huge amounts of online information. In the not-too-distant future, many physicians will carry portable computers to help them at the bedside, and individual medical records will be posted on the Internet with links to pertinent articles. Information specialists will be needed to help organize and maintain the necessary databases.

The Internet, of course, is the fastest-growing information source on the planet. George M. Lundberg, M.D., former editor of *JAMA* [55, see Appendix A] and now editor-in-chief of Medscape [10], believes that the Internet will prove to be as significant in civilization's development as the invention of the printing press. Its effect on my own work has been phenomenal. In 1996, I launched the Quackwatch [28] site to provide readers of my *Consumer Health* textbook with full-text access to some of the book's citations. I also thought it would be useful to provide relevant news and additional source materials. I soon discovered that other sites, newsgroups, and email messages from visitors provided a wealth of valuable information—and that documents that had previously taken weeks or months to collect might be found within minutes using a search engine.

Information retrieval is both a science and an art. The science is in knowing *where* to search. The art involves *how* to search. This book contains practical pointers on both. The toughest aspect is judging reliability. General standards are easy to articulate. Everyone agrees, for example, that information should be evidence-based, and that citations from major peer-reviewed journals are a plus. But peer reviewers are not all equal, and MEDLINE [96] inclusion does not guarantee reliability. It's also possible to list signs of unreliability, as Quackwatch does in an article called "Signs of a Quacky Web Site." For example, sites that sell products or promote "alternative" methods are often untrustworthy. But no standard can substitute for expert medical knowledge. Top experts can not only assess what has been published, they also know what's happening in their field that has not yet been publicized.

In many cases, professional searchers can rely on their professional clients to judge the quality of what is found. In other situations, consultants can advise whether specific sources are reliable. It also helps to develop your own list of reliable sources. My "short list" includes:

For professionals:
Medical Matrix [8] (peer-reviewed gateway to medical sites)
Medscape (news and an electronic medical journal)
The Medical Letter on Drugs and Therapeutics [58]
Journal of the American Medical Association
New England Journal of Medicine [61]

For consumers:
Consumer Reports on Health [47] (the best all-around newsletter for consumers)

FDA Consumer [88] (food and drug information in print and online)

CBSHealthwatch [17] (general health information)

Some observers hope that the Internet will develop a "certification" system analogous to the board certification of physicians. There are so many Web sites and content can change so frequently that I doubt whether any formal effort will succeed. Nevertheless, the highest-quality sites will rise above the crowd.

Exciting times lie ahead of us.

Stephen Barrett, M.D., a retired psychiatrist who lives in Allentown, Pennsylvania, is a prominent author, editor, and consumer advocate. His 47 books include *The Health Robbers: A Close Look at Quackery in America*, *The Vitamin Pushers: How the Health Food Industry Is Selling America a Bill of Goods*, and five editions of the college textbook *Consumer Health: A Guide to Intelligent Decisions*. Dr. Barrett is board chairman of Quackwatch, Inc., and a board member of the National Council Against Health Fraud. He operates three Web sites: Quackwatch (www.quackwatch.com), Chirobase (www.chirobase.org), and MLM Watch (www.mlmwatch.org). He is reachable at (610) 437-1795 or sbinfo@quackwatch.com.

Acknowledgments

Without people to interview, there would be no book. Without incredibly warm, friendly, knowledgeable, generous people to interview, this book would not have been worth writing. And so, to Barbara, Fran, Tom, Peg, Auburn, Nancy, Alan, Pam, John, and Bonnie, a very deep thank you. Our conversations taught me so much more than mere searching techniques.

Again, without people to interview, there would be no book. I owe many thanks to the individuals who led me to these generous souls. Thanks go to Debora (Ralf) Shaw, Linda Cooper, and Reva Basch, for suggesting interviewees, and a very special thanks to the members of the medical librarians' listserv, who came through when I asked for their input on Super Searchers. Each day, I read the list and learn more and more from you dedicated professionals.

Perhaps the only problem with the fact that Reva Basch wrote the first two Super Searcher books and edits this series is that she, herself, cannot be interviewed. She knows the ins and outs of searching and knows how to put it into plain English. Thank you, Reva, for putting up with my "new author terrors," gently amending my writing, and convincing me that you really wanted me to do this book.

Thanks are also due to my friend John Bryans, editor-in-chief, who took the time to explain the process, discuss my concerns, and look at photos of my kids. For several years, we have looked for ways to work together on a project. I'm glad this is the one we found.

Patty Shannon at the Work Station transcribed each and every interview in this book. I am amazed at how easily she picked up the obscure medical terminology and grateful for the humorous comments she interjected into some of those 42-page transcripts. Janet Spavlik at Information Today efficiently handled everything that needed to be handled, sending books, papers, photos, and files to their respective destinations.

But my most important acknowledgment goes to my family. These are the people who ground me, balance my life, and let me know what's really important. Thank you, John; thank you, Ann; and especially, thank you, Mark. You are my rock.

Introduction

When Reva Basch and John Bryans first invited me to do a book in the *Super Searchers* series, I ran the gamut of emotions. I was flattered, enthusiastic, scared, and overwhelmed. After all, Reva is one of the "brand name" participants in the information field, and the other Super Searcher authors are professional colleagues whom I've looked up to for several years.

What I didn't anticipate was just how humbled I would be by these interviews with top medical searchers. The men and women in this book are different from most of the searchers I have met. Sure, they all enjoy the thrill of the hunt and the wordplay associated with text searching, but there's an added fillip to their dedication. Each one of these searchers treats his or her work as a mission. Perhaps Barbara Bernoff Cavanaugh said it best when I asked her what makes a good medical searcher:

"Believing that what you do is important. It's different from other kinds of research, because sometimes it really can be life and death issues that you're dealing with. You have to be someone who's willing to exhaust all the possibilities before determining that you can stop. With medicine, it's often not a matter of finding the answer, it's a matter of finding different perspectives on the topics, so that physicians or end users can get different viewpoints and make their own interpretations."

Life and death issues. That certainly is different from other kinds of searching. Pam Geyer reminded me that, no matter how much a product manager may believe his or her job is on the line based on the results of a search, working with a patient who has just been told he or she has cancer is what brings you back to reality.

The Internet is affecting almost all aspects of healthcare delivery. According to the Internet research firm Cyber Dialogue [161, see Appendix A], by mid-1999, 36 percent of all Internet users had searched for health and medical information online, and 3.4 million Americans had requested a particular drug from their doctors based on information they found on the Internet. Whole companies have sprung up to effect the delivery of medical goods from business to business and from business to consumer. Retail pharmacies, both virtual and "clicks & mortar," deliver medical advice on their Web sites, alongside shopping carts full of drugs and healthcare products. In its first year of existence, the eHealthCareWorld Trade Show [163] attracted 120 exhibitors and 4,500 attendees. Who has not seen a health news feature on television that ended with "for more details, see our Web site…"? Who hasn't heard of DrKoop.com [18]?

Yet this very accessibility to information and products has its own hazards. As I write this, organizations like HI-Ethics, Internet Healthcare Coalition, and Health on the Net are struggling with the issue of content reliability. Their members are working on healthcare Web site standards, in attempts to ensure at least some minimum accountability for accuracy, validity, timeliness, and consumer privacy. But we're not there yet, and even when standards are issued, there's no assurance that a particular site will adhere to them.

So, if you're a consumer, how do you tell good information from bad? Where do you go for reliable information in terms you can understand? If you're a medical professional, how do you cope with the patient who has been misinformed by a supposedly reliable Web site? How do you add searching and patient email to an already full day? If you're a research professional, how do you keep up with the profusion of new sources or choose a vendor for the traditional resources? How do you teach consumers that just because it's on the Internet doesn't mean it's true?

All these issues demand the attention of medical searchers. My underlying premise for this book was that highly trained and experienced medical searchers could guide us through the morass of healthcare information online. With their help, we would learn how to evaluate what's out there and how to select the best sources for the question at hand. In retrospect, these professionals have given us the perspective to do just that. They've also given us the insight to realize that, sometimes, we should leave it to the experts.

Selecting the interviewees for this book was a task that took several months. Many are not published writers or well-known speakers. They are not flashy about what they do. There's a saying within the medical profession that, when it comes to surgery, you don't necessarily want the doctor who writes about the subject, but rather the one who does the same procedure ten times a week. In some ways, finding medical Super Searchers was a similar process. While some of those who know their subjects inside and out write and speak brilliantly (and I interviewed several of them), others stay in their offices and libraries, quietly doing the work that makes their clients—the medical professionals—successful in *their* work. Finding these unsung heroes meant a lot of networking, using contacts built up through the years, and reading postings on the medical librarians' electronic mailing lists. I was looking for the searchers' searchers, and found them through the plaudits of their colleagues.

The men and women you meet in this book come from a wide range of backgrounds and bring a variety of experiences to the table. As a whole, they're a varied matrix of education, experiences, and employers. Those with medical degrees employ those degrees very differently when they wear their "searcher" hats. Those with library science degrees have taken different directions, combining the M.L.S. (Master's in Library Science) with other degrees and experiences to bring a special knowledge to their searching. Several don't have degrees in library science, but are self-taught searchers with deep subject expertise.

Although four work in a university setting, they differ greatly in their specialties and approaches to their subjects. One assists in reference work at a veterinary school and a nursing school, along with her work for the biomedical library. Another teaches physicians how to do their own searching. Her colleague at the same institution is a practicing physician who returned to school for his M.L.S. He assists his medical colleagues in their research and brings his professional knowledge to bear on the results. Also in the university setting, one interviewee works with public health issues, finding epidemiology statistics and evaluating healthcare Web sites for consumers and professionals.

One former medical school librarian is an independent researcher who works extensively in the nursing and allied health field, while at the same time assisting in public health issues. Another independent works with pharmaceutical and medical device manufacturers, attorneys, and their consultants. Yet another has based her entire business on directly serving those men and women who most benefit from quality medical information—the patients. Serving the patient is also the motive of another physician interviewee, who is part of a provider system and who moderates its online client information service.

Two interviewees with medical librarianship backgrounds took very different turns in their careers. Both now work for consulting firms; one searches toxicology issues, the other advises pharmaceutical companies on how to find the information they need to stay competitive.

Yet, despite their differences, some common themes appeared in interview after interview.

DEDICATION

First, I must repeat what I said at the beginning of this introduction: These professionals are dedicated to helping. They are very careful about what they do and are constantly aware that what they do impacts an individual's health. They don't usually think in the abstract about "healthcare"; rather, they talk in terms of "the patient," "the doctor," or "my client." When they work with consumers, they advise them to work with their own physicians, because each situation is different. No literature search compares with a personal visit to the doctor.

Many of the interviewees consider teaching to be a large part of their jobs. They speak in terms of passing on their knowledge to others and teaching doctors and nurses how to access clinical literature with the tools at hand. Even when they use sophisticated search tools at their own institutions, they are careful to teach medical students how to use the less-sophisticated systems that are ubiquitous on the Web. They believe that knowing how to use these systems to their best advantage will enable new doctors to find the literature they need, wherever they end up working. Searchers who work with consumers teach them how to present search results to their doctors without cutting off the lines of communication. They teach their clients how to approach medical professionals as partners. In short, they *teach*.

RELIANCE ON PROVEN SOURCES

Despite all the changes in healthcare delivery, medical searching still relies to a great extent on databases, which have existed for decades. When it comes to clinical medicine, the National Library of Medicine's MEDLINE [96] has no peer. The MEDLINE filees have been avilable from 1966, and researchers still swear by it for basic, peer-reviewed references. The September 1999 demise of ELHILL, the direct-to-the-source, command-language version of MEDLINE, provoked eulogies among several of the searchers. Two were prepared to hold a wake in its memory.

Depending on the question, a handful of other databases typically are added to the search. There's a lot of commonality here. When it comes to scientific research in the medical literature, searchers agree on the "Big Three": MEDLINE, EMBASE [131], and BIOSIS [123]. One searcher went a step further and added

SciSearch [147], for its time-sensitive coverage of scientific meetings and conferences.

For nursing and allied health, there's only one place to start: CINAHL [127]. Developed by and for auxiliary health professionals, CINAHL was cited for its in-depth coverage of patient care. Surprisingly, ERIC [132] was also cited as particularly good for the allied health professions. Traditionally, we think of ERIC as an education database, but that is precisely why it covers the exceptional needs of young patients very well. Similarly, when it comes to the psychosocial aspects of illness, PsycLIT [146] is a frequently used source.

"Pipeline information," that is, what's coming down the pipe from research and development at drug and device manufacturers, is important to many in the medical field. Despite the profusion of commercial pipeline sites on the World Wide Web, there's still no adequate substitute for the pharmaceutical and device databases from ADIS [43], PJB [65], and F-D-C Reports [53]. Drug and device companies need these databases to stay competitive. The companies that produce these databases conduct proactive research into manufacturers' pipelines, making them superior to their Web-based counterparts.

PRECISION

At a time when natural language searching is gaining popularity, and even professional searchers embrace text-word or free-text searching in full-text databases, the medical world stands firm as a holdout against the trend. It's not surprising that medical Super Searchers are precision searchers. They have to be. So many diseases, disorders, and drugs masquerade under different identities that searchers must use controlled vocabulary terms to be sure of getting all the variations. The tree-structure indexes of systems like MEDLINE and CINAHL allow searchers to move up and down the ladders to find the precise aspect of the disorder they're looking for. Most of the searchers use hedges or templates to keep them from forgetting some key aspect of a search. They warn that not being aware of the difference between a disorder and its medical specialty—searching on gastrointestinal disorders instead of gastroenterology—can leave the novice searcher with no results.

Yet, despite their focus on methodical searching, medical Super Searchers are quite aware of the limitations of controlled vocabularies. When a new treatment or newly discovered disease hits the news, there is no precise way to look for it. It hasn't been around long enough for the indexing to become codified. That's when the searchers turn to text-word searching. Text-word is also the best way to find the right terminology when your requestor has given you a lay term to start with.

EVIDENCE-BASED MEDICINE

Evidence-based medicine, or EBM, was the topic of considerable discussion among the searchers interviewed in this book. EBM refers to the process of searching medical literature in order to find controlled clinical trials that can be applied to a particular patient. In essence, it is medicine based on scientific data that can be replicated.

Yet, as favorable as this is for most clinical situations, it is not always appropriate. EBM isn't adequate in a research situation, when the requestor needs every single instance in which a drug is used, clinical trial or not. It's not sufficient when a patient has an unusual cluster of symptoms, which has only been written up in a single case report. EBM also took some flack from searchers for being too narrow in its focus, preventing researchers from seeing the larger picture which might lie outside the arena of controlled clinical trials.

Prior to these interviews, I'd had only cursory contact with the concept of evidence-based medicine. I deliberately retained several different definitions in the interviews, to illustrate the varying

views of how important EBM is to medical searching and to the
practice of clinical medicine.

ALTERNATIVE MEDICINE

With the current interest in herbal and nontraditional medicine, it was natural to ask expert searchers how they find authoritative information on alternative medicine. It was a bit like asking
how porcupines make love. The answer is, "Very carefully."
Sources for what we term "alternative" or "complementary" medicine are universally viewed as less authoritative than sources for
mainstream medicine. There is no information source with even a
fraction of the stature of MEDLINE. There are very few controlled
clinical trials; each scientific study of an alternative treatment
must be reviewed on its own merits. Searchers can't decide on the
validity of a particular study by looking at its source; alternative
medicine has neither a single peer-reviewed database nor a journal. Muddying the waters even further are retail Web sites that
provide supposedly valid medical information, couched in pseudo-scientific terms, for the apparent purpose of selling the herb of
the month.

KEEPING UP WITH THE WEB

These Super Searchers were in total agreement that the
Internet is vital to their efforts. Yet you wouldn't know it by their
unaided recall. When asked about sources, almost every single
professional searcher immediately talked about traditional databases. It wasn't until deeper into our conversations that they
brought up Web-based resources. It seemed almost as if they
were still not comfortable acknowledging the Web as a valuable
resource. Yet, in each interview, the Internet emerged as an
invaluable asset in answering almost any question. Epidemiology
statistics have never been easier to find; access to government
publications is simplified; association documents are readily

accessible. Manufacturers publish their Materials Safety Data Sheets on the Web; terminology that hasn't yet been codified can be tested in free searches. Electronic mailing lists offer ways to network and learn about new sources. Individual journals offer current-awareness services on topics of choice. The complete contents of classic textbooks are available in full on the Web.

Accompanying the wonderland of the Internet is the frustration that so much is new and changing. There's no way to keep up with it all. We're each like the Red Queen, running as fast as we can just to keep from falling behind. Super Searchers' methods of keeping up are so similar as to be almost parrot-like: Talk to other searchers and share new Web sites. Maintain an organized set of bookmarks. Read the professional journals. Read topic-specific literature. Participate in a mailing list or discussion group. Get frustrated and fall behind.

I was particularly pleased that each interviewee considers talking to other searchers and sharing their knowledge to be basic requirements of the job. While, almost universally, they consider too many electronic mailing lists distracting, most find at least one that is useful to their work. Basic to human knowledge is the need to share.

Unfortunately, it would be logistically impossible for each reader of this book to meet each interviewee. Instead, I introduce them to you in the pages that follow. I hope I asked them the questions that you would have asked.

I must admit that I struggled with the order in which to present these conversations. I begin with the classic, medical university librarian, setting the stage for the variations that follow. So the first four interviews bring you three views of medical school librarianship followed by an independent researcher whose work is heavily devoted to auxiliary health professionals.

I then move from searchers who work with medical professionals to two who work in public health and public safety. These are followed by two who work directly with patients—in distinctly different ways. I end with two interviewees who work closely with manufacturers of medical devices and pharmaceuticals.

To keep from cluttering the interviews with URLs and footnotes, I have prepared an appendix of resources mentioned in the interviews. The first time a resource is cited in an interview, it is accompanied by its reference number in the appendix. The appendix is divided into Web resources, print, and email contacts. I have also prepared a glossary of terms specific to the online searching world of medicine and healthcare, with a few clinical terms thrown in. I've made no attempt to be comprehensive; that would be impossible in such a limited space. However, I hope that handy access to this selective glossary will help alleviate any confusion brought on by the specialized terms used in this book.

I am still in awe of the men and women you will meet in the following pages and am profoundly grateful to them for their willingness to talk with me. All of them gave a lot of their time to share the tips and tricks that they've learned through experience. They've spent many years working with healthcare sources, learning to extract just what they need and to weed out the rest. Whether you read these interviews in sequence or open the book at random, I'm sure you'll find tools worth adding to your own armamentarium.

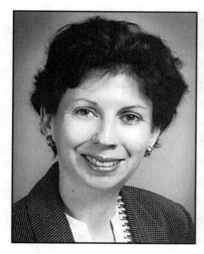

Barbara Bernoff Cavanaugh

Life Science Generalist

Barbara Bernoff Cavanaugh, M.L.S., is Liaison for the Biomedical, Veterinary and Dental Libraries and Ovid Databases Coordinator at the University of Pennsylvania Biomedical Library in Philadelphia.

bbc@pobox.upenn.edu

Barbara, your title is quite a mouthful. How did you get so immersed in the life sciences?

I actually fell into the life sciences aspect of librarianship. I was an English major in college and met a medical librarian in my senior year. Her work doing research in the medical field sounded genuinely interesting and very important to me. With my humanities background, though, I didn't necessarily want to settle into the medical side of things. Then I fell into a job at Pennsylvania Hospital through an archives practicum that I was taking and really developed a love for the medical literature.

What are you doing now?

I remember my first day of work back in 1980. Someone asked to see *Harrison's* [39, see Appendix A], and I responded "Harrison's what?" I didn't know he meant *Harrison's Principles of Internal Medicine,* which is the bible of internal medicine. I was half-amused, half-put-off by journal titles such as *Gut, Blood* and *Brain.* I thought, "Where have I landed? What kind of a world is this?" Somehow, I have gone from that to routinely teaching classes with medical literature and medical jargon. The funniest example I have is in the context of explaining MEDLINE's [96] Explode function. I was in a group advising the class to "Explode the male genitalia," and I didn't even think about what I was saying until someone in the audience cringed. I guess I've come a long way from my English major days!

To answer your question more directly, I'm a reference librarian at the University of Pennsylvania Biomedical Library, and I rotate to the Veterinary and Dental libraries as well. Both of these smaller libraries have professional librarians, but I work with them on training and special projects, reference work, instruction, and so forth.

Are there many differences among the three libraries either in subject matter or in how you search?

The main difference is cultural. The biomedical library is larger, and a lot of the reference transactions are done at a busy reference desk. You have less time to find the answer or help someone with a question, unless you schedule time for a lengthier consultation away from the reference desk. In the smaller settings, it's more personal. There's no reference desk *per se*, you work in a more relaxed manner, and you can usually go into much more depth. As for searching, there are specific tricks and techniques for using the databases that vary according to the specific subject matter, but the basic approaches are the same.

What a great segue. What is the basic approach that you use?

We tend to be very MEDLINE-centric, so most searches will begin with MEDLINE. We use the Ovid [158] version, because we like the search engine very much. We'll supplement that with a search of the National Library of Medicine's free version of MEDLINE, PubMed [112], which has extremely current pre-MEDLINE citations. However, it's really, really important not to limit any search to just that one database. Generally, we take a search to BIOSIS [123] from there; you get a lot of meeting abstracts and conference proceedings, and even some book chapter information that would be missing from MEDLINE. Often, we go to the ISI Citation Indexes [140] online, which we use to supplement for scope and more currency than MEDLINE. So, to be thorough, we would want to check at least that variety of databases. If it's nursing-related, we would search CINAHL [127], the nursing database, as well.

What about in the veterinary library; would that basic lineup of MEDLINE-BIOSIS-ISI-PubMed-CINAHL change?

The major database for veterinary literature is CAB Abstracts [124], produced in Britain by CAB International. It covers the veterinary journals more extensively than MEDLINE. MEDLINE only covers about 75 vet journals, and CAB Abstracts covers hundreds. It also covers related literature, such as animal production, agriculture, and the broader life sciences. In fact, I think BIOSIS and CAB cover all of medicine more broadly than MEDLINE does. MEDLINE tries to be selective and specific to peer-reviewed journals, whereas these other databases try to be broad and comprehensive. BIOSIS is very important. BIOSIS sometimes picks up a meeting abstract or proceeding that CAB misses, or vice versa. There's not complete overlap in coverage on that kind of ephemeral information. The other important database is AGRICOLA [81], from the National Agricultural Library. That is the only source for National Agricultural Library information, which is not included in the other databases.

One thing that you have to be aware of when you're using MEDLINE for veterinary medicine is that the "veterinary" subheading excludes animal studies. A broader approach would be to limit the search to "animal."

What databases would you add to MEDLINE for dental?

Fortunately, MEDLINE covers all the dental journals. Even so, it's important to remember that you can combine a general subject with the exploded MeSH heading "mouth diseases" or "dentistry," to be more comprehensive. In Ovid, you can limit a search to dental journals.

When I started working with the dental library, I learned that a lot of dental research is much broader than the general public might expect, particularly regarding bone research, a lot of biochemical and nutrition research, and even AIDS research. So it's often necessary to go beyond the clinical information in MEDLINE. We still check BIOSIS and ISI for conference-type information and life science information.

All the databases I've named, except ISI, we access through Ovid, so users and librarians can rerun the search from one to the other, all within the same interface.

A single interface enhances the search process?

A single interface makes it easier to figure out what search techniques work best. Part of the problem with having to use a different interface or search engine is that it's very important to get to know how each search engine works in order to get good results. So when you're in PubMed, you're going to use a very different technique than when you search the Ovid version of MEDLINE. Even within Ovid's array of databases, searching MEDLINE versus CAB versus BIOSIS, you need to use different techniques. So, the more common ground between interfaces, the better.

What's a typical question in the biomedical library?

Someone recently came to the reference desk wanting information on tendon ruptures in the gluteus medius. That turned out to be an extremely specific kind of question where we found very little information. It's frustrating to do this type of research at the reference desk where you have so little time with a person, especially a clinician who needs to rush back to the floor. Having to do these things in split seconds poses extra challenges.

Do you have an opportunity to do a reference interview there?

Yes. It has to be very quick and to the point, though. My favorite question to ask is, "What are you looking for specifically?" Usually the initial presentation of the question is broad, or they try to simplify or generalize it in some way. If you just start off with the information they give you, you can waste a lot of time going off in the wrong direction. Typically, they'll ask, "Where do I go for information on tendon ruptures?", when what they really want is a very specific tendon. Information on tendon ruptures in general would not have been satisfactory. So asking them to restate it often helps a lot.

Sometimes I feel like the attorney in the movie *Philadelphia* who says, "now explain it to me like I'm a six-year-old." Even if I think I understand, I say, "Well, this topic's a little out of my subject knowledge, can you explain it to me in simple terms?" Because I'm not a medical professional, I sometimes need a more simple explanation so that I understand what I'm looking for and it's not just jargon. It also forces patrons to think through what they really want as they articulate their question.

When somebody comes to you with a very broad question, does that change your reference interview?

Yes, we usually make sure that they really want it that broad. I will follow up and ask "What particular aspects of that topic are you interested in?" or "This topic in relation to what?" If it's something clinical, I might ask if there's a gender- or age-group-specific aspect.

Sometimes, rather than looking for something specific, they're writing a book chapter or a review article. Then they do want all the information on a topic. Someone recently wanted information on the history of orthopedics.

Since Persia, perhaps?

I think it was just the United States, so that put a time limit on it. Actually, that kind of question is fairly easy to cover in MED-LINE. There's a "history" subheading, which this patron and his research assistants hadn't used. He was very pleased and said that I had found in three minutes what he had spent weeks looking for, all because they didn't know that simple tactic in MEDLINE.

On the medical side, do you ever use hard copy sources?

Yes, if I need to get a broad overview or understanding of a subject before I go online. Sometimes, the patron is just looking for very basic information. That would be like looking for a needle in a haystack in a database like MEDLINE, which is mostly research on very specific kinds of topics. If they just want basic information on a particular disease, or an overview, it's better to send them to a textbook.

At Penn, you mainly use Ovid to get at your information. Any tips or tricks for getting the most out of it?

For MEDLINE, I have some very important tips. You definitely get better results if you do use MeSH, the subject heading structure. Sometimes you need to combine a MeSH heading with a keyword if it's a newer topic that doesn't have a suitable MeSH heading. Two of my favorite examples of that, which I stole from a colleague, are "spiral CT" and "functional MRI." Subject headings exist for "computed tomography" and "magnetic resonance imaging," but not for those specific types. So, if you search on a subject heading and combine it with the keyword "spiral" or "functional," you get very good results; a keyword search or a MeSH heading search alone would not yield good results.

With MEDLINE, it's important not to confuse diseases with medical specialties. I had someone in a class once who worked in gastrointestinal diseases. She was always typing "gastroenterology" to combine it with other topics, and would end up with zero hits. That's because "gastroenterology" will retrieve articles on the practice of gastroenterology as a medical profession; it won't retrieve gastrointestinal diseases, which is a separate subject heading. If you want diseases, you have to search that actual heading instead. That's a very common mistake. People will type in "geriatrics" and retrieve articles about the profession, when they really want something else entirely.

They actually want a subject, and then the age as a limit?

Right. They should be searching for a disease and then limiting to an age group, rather than using "geriatrics" as a subject term. The same is true for "children" or "elderly," which people commonly try to use as search terms. If you use MEDLINE's limit function, which gives you a very neat breakdown of age groups, you get much better retrieval. Ovid facilitates use of those types of limits in MEDLINE.

Another tip is to not confuse viruses or organisms with the infections they cause. A common mistake that people make is to search "HIV" when they really mean AIDS or HIV infections. You'll get totally different results with those different subject headings. You also have to be careful not to confuse symptoms with diseases, for example, "depression" versus "depressive disorder."

For databases that don't have such a highly refined thesaurus structure with such a wide range of limit options, we teach people to use a lot of synonyms and truncation. For BIOSIS or CAB, we advise them to string out a search like "dog or dogs or canine" and combine that with "lyme or lymes or borrelia"—borrelia is the agent that causes Lyme disease. I would truncate "borrelia" after the "l" to get other varieties of word endings. We have to teach when to truncate and when to actually spell out the plural, but it's very, very important to use synonyms and truncation in those databases or you will miss a lot.

Another general tip for all the databases is to string out your separate concepts on different search lines. I force myself to do that, even if I'm in a hurry or feel like I know exactly what I need. On one line, you have "dog or dogs or canine," and your next search set has "lyme or lymes or borrelia." Then you combine the two. That's so important because it encourages you to try other combinations if that first search doesn't yield good results. If you string it all out on one line, you need to retype everything all over again to try something else, and it can seem too tedious to users to have to keep doing that.

That's one of my frustrations with Web-based search engines. You usually can't do iterative searching.

Exactly. One of Ovid's strengths, which is unique for a Web-based interface, is that it lets you build a search history and go on and on without a limit to how many search sets you can create. It lets you combine and try different things. That's really the art of searching—trying lots of different combinations. Something like PubMed, which end users initially like because it is so easy, has an excellent relevancy engine that works behind the scenes. Users don't have to think about anything. They can type in a search without thinking about the strategy and still get good hits. The problem is that they're not encouraged to try to revise it in any way or to think it through beyond that.

Ovid presents you with tree structures and subheadings so that you can think through your topic. It even lets you browse a permuted index. Sometimes Ovid's mapping won't bring you to the best term, but if you browse the permuted index you can get ideas for other subject headings that you might not have thought of.

PubMed allows some browsing now, too. It also has a "related article" button, but, in my opinion, it takes you off track. You lose the initial thread you were following and go off on another "related article" thread. If you're trying to be systematic and thorough, you can begin to lose pieces of your search.

I think PubMed is going to become more and more popular, though, since they plan to broaden the scope to include life sciences and to include actual primary research reports in its PubMed Central. They're going to make the database linkable to more and more full-text information.

How delightful to be able to just hyperlink to the full text!

Exactly. In fact, I think that's the main area of competition among vendors in life sciences—how to link the bibliographic databases to full text. It's interesting to watch organizations like Ovid and the National Institutes of Health [102] going off in different directions, trying to link full text to the databases. Ovid's been a leader in that. They offer hundreds of full-text journals, so you can link from MEDLINE and read a full-text article. Most medical schools seem to use Ovid as their system of choice. Companies like ISI and its Web of Science [140] product do something very different. They actually allow linkage to publishers' Web sites and journals. So if Penn, for example, subscribes electronically to Academic Press journals, we can link to those journals right from within the ISI citation indexes. ISI doesn't package the journal access, they're just facilitating that linkage.

Ovid, on the other hand, is trying to aggregate the full text, actually selling access to the journals and reformatting the journals in SGML. There are pros and cons to both approaches. Ovid's approach allows more linkage. You can link from the references to the text of the article, or from the references to MEDLINE citations, and you just have one source for the journals. With ISI's approach, you can see the journals in Acrobat format (PDF), which users like because it looks like the print journal, and the libraries can negotiate individually with publishers for subscriptions.

Also, Ovid now facilitates linking to publisher Web sites, which shows that both trends are in demand. There are definite pros and cons to each, and it remains to be seen which will become the more popular avenue.

A lot of information that used to be available only to professionals is now on consumer-oriented Web sites. What's your opinion of that?

At Penn, we do get some consumer-level requests from patients using the Hospital of the University of Pennsylvania or the other affiliated hospitals in the area. We also get people from the community who just come in, and we get phone calls from consumers all over the country.

In general, having PubMed free online is revolutionizing the availability of medical information. But it can be confusing for consumers because there's so much out there. That's the real challenge on the Web—filtering out the good consumer health information from the poor information. That's not new, though; even with some of the traditional consumer health magazines, it's a challenge. They'll run an article on the benefits of a new vitamin, strategically placed next to an ad for that vitamin. You see similar things on the Web. You need to ask yourself who's producing this and what their motives are.

On the other hand, I think it's wonderful that information is so readily available for consumers, because it's important that they try to become educated and ask questions of their doctors. Early in my career, I started and developed the *Consumer Health and Nutrition Index*, which Oryx Press continued for about ten years. So consumer health is one of my favorite topics.

What do you think makes a good medical searcher?

Believing that what you do is important. It's different from other kinds of research, because sometimes it really can be life and death issues that you're dealing with. You have to be someone who's willing to exhaust all the possibilities before determining that you can stop. With medicine, it's often not a matter of finding the answer, it's a matter of finding different perspectives on the topics, so that physicians or end users can get different viewpoints and make their own interpretations.

A personal interest in the subject matter is important. Even though I don't have a medical background, I've always been interested in health and have read a lot in that area. When I'm searching, I'm interested in the results that I'm finding, which encourages me to keep looking.

It's important to look in unexpected places. Even if you think that you've covered all the important databases, it doesn't hurt to look somewhere else. You'd be surprised what might turn up in an unexpected location, either on the Web or in a database that's not directly related to your subject.

How do you keep up with the field? Are new sources coming out for the professional researcher?

Within medicine, there aren't that many new databases, but the proliferation of information on the Web is really hard to keep up with. The short answer to your question is that I don't keep up with it. I don't think it's possible. It's more important to communicate—constantly—with your peers. I'm very lucky at Penn; I have really, really knowledgeable colleagues with specific areas of expertise—whether it's dental or vet or nursing or life sciences—and we always draw upon each other's areas of knowledge. But finding information is mostly serendipity, and then remembering to log it away for a time when you might need it.

How do you keep track of what you've logged away?

I'm not entirely successful at that. I keep a lot of bookmarks, but it's time-consuming to organize them. Every now and then, I'll drag things around and put them in folders.

We at Penn maintain Web pages in the different subject specialties, so we've created our own Yahoo! [153], if you will. Someone using our home page [173] can click on "Web Resources" and see a breakdown for life sciences, dental, vet, government resources, statistical resources, nursing, and so on. The library staff is always adding to these pages, which helps us keep up. When we do stumble upon something, we add it to the appropriate page.

Do you think the information on the Web is actually different from the information we used to get through other sources, or is it just repackaged?

It's a bit of both. Someone was looking for physicians' starting salaries, and the American Medical Association told her to look in a certain publication that we have in the library. Another librarian and I, along with the patron, scoured this book, and could not find physicians' starting salaries. Just to see what would happen, I went to AltaVista [149], did a keyword search, and instantly found a Web site that had a beautiful chart with that information. I think that's an example of repackaging, where information that we used to assume we would only find in a directory was put up on the Web by another organization. But a lot of the information is different, such as new kinds of research that you wouldn't have heard about beforehand. It's a combination of the two.

The general search engines have their uses. I often find that a comprehensive search engine such as AltaVista will find documents buried in a Web site, even if that Web site's own search engine doesn't locate them.

Where do you think it's all going?

That's exciting to think about. The definite trend is toward integration. All the vendors are clearly competing to integrate the databases through multi-file searching and de-duping, linking to full text, and linking to document ordering. I think we're going to see more and more integration down the line. What the NIH is doing with the PubMed Central product is a good example. I can't really speculate on what it means for medical journals—whether print versions will still exist down the line or not. Right now, we can't imagine not having print editions of some of those titles, even though we have them electronically. Instead of substituting, we're still duplicating at this point.

Librarians worry about archiving; if they drop their print subscription or change the source of their electronic access, what guarantee do they have of continued access to the archives? Companies like Ovid assure their users that they recognize the importance of continued access. But it's still frightening because it's so intangible; there is concern over who "owns" the archives, especially if they are accessed remotely. What happens if the online journal providers undergo changes?

What's the role of the librarian in the future?

One role will be a greater responsibility in facilitating access to synthesized information—that is, meta-analysis—which is an important trend in medicine right now. I still see the role of librarian as organizing and facilitating access to data. We'll see more and more instruction, education, and training users to do these things for themselves. In medicine, the days are gone when the librarians do the search and send the results to the user. So much information is available directly to the user. The most important thing we can do right now is give users the skills and education they need to search for it effectively.

Super Searcher Power Tips

➤ On the benefits of a uniform interface

A single interface makes it easier to figure out what search techniques work best. The more common ground between interfaces, the better.

➤ On fine-tuning the reference interview

My favorite question is, "What are you looking for specifically?" Sometimes, I feel like the attorney in the movie *Philadelphia*, when he says, "Now explain it to me like I'm a six-year-old." It also forces patrons to think through what they really want as they articulate their questions.

➤ On the value of not going online

Sometimes, the patron is just looking for some very basic information. That would be like looking for a needle in a haystack in a database like MEDLINE. If they just want basic information on a particular disease or an overview, it's better to send them to a textbook.

➤ On combining MeSH with free-text

Sometimes, you need to combine a MeSH heading with a keyword if it's a newer topic that doesn't have a suitable MeSH heading. If you search on the broad subject heading and combine it with a more specific keyword, you often get very good results, whereas a keyword search or a MeSH heading search alone would not yield good results.

➤ On selecting the right MeSH headings

It's important not to confuse diseases with medical specialties, or viruses or organisms with the infections that they cause. You also have to be careful not to confuse symptoms with diseases, for example, "depression" versus "depressive disorder."

➤ On the value of truncation

For databases like BIOSIS or CAB that don't have a highly refined thesaurus structure with a wide range of limit options, use a lot of synonyms and truncation. It's very, very important to do that, or you will miss a lot.

➤ On separating the search into separate strings

I string out my separate concepts on different search lines—"dog or dogs or canine," and the next search set would have "lyme or lymes or borrelia"—and then combine the two. That encourages you to try other combinations if that first search doesn't yield good results. If you string it all out on one line, you need to retype everything to try something else, and it can seem too tedious to keep doing that.

➤ On using a general search engine

The general search engines have their uses. I often find that a comprehensive search engine such as AltaVista will find documents buried in a Web site, even if that Web site's own search engine doesn't locate them.

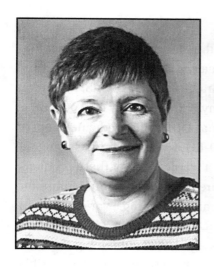

Frances A. Brahmi

Educating Future Physicians

Frances A. Brahmi, M.L.S., is Acting Director of the Ruth Lilly Medical Library at Indiana University in Indianapolis.

fbrahmi@iupui.edu

Fran, could you tell me a bit about what you do and how you ended up doing it?

I've been here for over 20 years, beginning as a reference librarian and search analyst. As time went on, my responsibility increased and my interest changed from being a reference librarian and searcher to a teacher and participant in the medical curriculum. I've become more of a medical educator than a medical librarian.

Who are your patrons?

The library primarily serves the faculty, students, and staff of the medical school, the nursing school, and the school of allied health. Then, in varying degrees, we help anyone who comes into the library. All Indiana citizens are free to come in and use our collection, but we have a variable scale in terms of what we charge our primary versus our secondary users.

You wrote an article comparing the many different versions of MEDLINE [96, see Appendix A]. Can you go into that a bit for me?

I started searching back in the early '80s, and around 1986 end-user systems started appearing. The National Library of Medicine [103] came out with Grateful Med [91]. BRS, which was a big medical database company, introduced its own version of end-user searching. The National Library of Medicine licensed various companies to create CD-ROM-based products using the MEDLINE database. There was a whole flurry of these products. So, when we were trying to figure out how we should jump into the end user market, I looked at and compared a variety of them. The article that I published in *MD Computing* [57] looked at how the different vendors were massaging and enhancing the same data to make it more accessible or, sometimes, not so accessible. I constructed search strategies to test the various interfaces on how they handled certain questions. I looked at their list of stop words. How did they handle searching for "interleukin 1, 2, 3, 8"? How did they handle "stage IV carcinoma"?

The way a database is constructed makes a big difference in what the user gets out of it. It was very interesting to look at the various products on the market that were all MEDLINE, but either consisted of subsets of the data or handled the data in different ways, making the output very dissimilar.

Are any of those products still on the market?

Grateful Med still is, for sure. It has gone through many, many versions, and is now Internet-accessible and free from NLM's Web page. PubMed [112] and Grateful Med are two ways of getting at the same information, but using very different interfaces. Grateful Med is still a viable product, and PubMed is almost a household word by now.

What are the ramifications of MEDLINE being accessible in so many different forms?

It's a great development, not only for consumers but for researchers as well. The fact that MEDLINE has become so ubiquitous is forcing us all to look at the resources we use in a more critical way. In teaching medical students, I tell them they need to know about information resources like the Web or MEDLINE not only for their own work, but because their patients will be coming to them with information they got off the Web. They need to be aware of these resources and be able to evaluate them. They have to be able to point out to their patients whether this is a good source of information, or not really authoritative, and to suggest that perhaps another Web site would be better.

Where do you send your students for MEDLINE?

We train them on the Ovid [158] version of MEDLINE that we have here in the library. In my opinion, Ovid is the best MED-LINE interface available right now. However, because we know that they may not always have Ovid at their fingertips, we also train them on PubMed. That way, no matter where they go, as long as they have an Internet connection they can get to MED-LINE. We train them on ways of manipulating the MEDLINE database so they can retrieve evidence-based-medicine-type articles from MEDLINE.

Can you give me a good lay definition of evidence-based medicine?

There are several definitions, but I like to think of evidence-based medicine as the way good physicians have always practiced medicine. They rely on their clinical skills combined with what they learn from the patient and from the literature. It's a combination of those three components and determining what the best evidence is as it relates to the patient. The difficulty in our day and age is that the literature component has become so vast that finding those two or three relevant articles, out of the more than nine million records in the MEDLINE database, is very challenging. That's the key to evidence-based medicine: How do you find the best evidence, based on good science and well-designed research, with a clinical result that you can apply to this patient? That's what we try to teach our students.

Here at Indiana University School of Medicine, the library faculty is responsible for a week-long clerkship that's required of all fourth-year medical students. During that week, we introduce the students to the concepts of evidence-based medicine: what it is, why it's important, and how you get at those evidence-based articles within MEDLINE. One session is devoted to critically appraising therapy and diagnosis articles.

What do you teach them?

We're teaching them that the key to finding clinical information is to first formulate your question. This question has four parts: Who is the patient, what is the intervention of interest, what "gold standard" are you comparing it to, and what outcome are you looking for? This approach was developed at McMaster University in Hamilton, Ontario [166]. We have saved search strategies developed at McMaster that students can plug into any MEDLINE search that has to do with diagnosis, therapy, prognosis, or etiology. We got the strategies from a wonderful book, *Evidence-Based Medicine: How to Practice and Teach EBM (Evidence-Based Medicine)* [187], by David L. Sackett, W. Scott Richardson, William Rosenberg, and R. Brian Haynes.

Have you modified those questions at all?

No, not really. They were developed by going through thousands of searches. They did clinical research to determine the strategies, which are based on lots of checking and re-checking, asking the question, doing the search, and seeing if they got comprehensive retrieval. The strategies are two-fold: You can search for diagnosis in a very precise way, or in a manner that will get you a larger output. The strategies vary, and determine whether you'll get a specific or a more general output.

Are all the concepts and descriptors included?

All the descriptors are in the saved strategy, but searchers need to find their own concepts. However, Ovid automatically maps a concept to the MeSH term. That's why we like it so much. You put in a term and it maps you to MeSH. If it can't find an exact match, it will give you a menu of close matches to choose from.

Do the McMaster templates work in PubMed?

Yes. In fact, the templates are available through PubMed, where they're called "Clinical Queries." If you click on Clinical Queries on PubMed's home page, it takes you to these hedges that I'm talking about—the four aspects of clinical medicine.

Would you suggest that consumers try this approach as well, or would you have some caveats about that?

I think consumers could be taught how to do this. After all, we're all after the same thing: "What is the best evidence out there? Is there a randomized controlled trial for the drug that I'm interested in?" or whatever.

In the four-part McMaster template, you used the phrase "gold standard." How would you define a gold standard? Where would a gold standard come from?

"Gold standard" comes from clinical practice itself; it's what the medical community has agreed is the best practice for diagnosing a particular disease entity or treating a particular affliction. Sometimes they're reflected in clinical practice guidelines, which are available directly from various professional associations. They are also reflected in NIH Consensus Guidelines [105], and AHCPR [80](Agency for Health Care Policy and Research, now known as Agency for Healthcare Research and Quality) guidelines.

One of my favorite sources for guidelines is MD Consult [6]. It gives you access to a lot of guidelines in one place.

Exactly. I think MD Consult is a wonderful service for physicians, I recommend it highly. It gives you full-text access to many of the articles cited in MEDLINE, as well as to many full-text books.

Do you ever see a role for case studies or case reports in evidence-based medicine?

Yes, because you won't always find a randomized controlled trial. It's important to know what's available, and to know the weaknesses and strengths of various study designs, but for certain questions a randomized controlled trial will not exist. There may be ethical or practical reasons. So, yes, there's room for all kinds of study designs, as long as you know what you're looking at, and that the results may be based on a non-controlled study design and may have a limited application. But case reports are still a place to start.

When are you finished with a search? How do you know how much time to spend on it?

That depends on the person I'm doing the search for. If I'm searching for a student who's doing a term paper, I'm finished in just a few minutes; if I get 25 good hits, that will be it. If I'm working for a researcher who's writing a comprehensive review article about a topic, I may take days. The depth and coverage that my user wants dictates how much time I spend on it. Then, when the same articles start popping up no matter what search strategy or databases I've used, I'm pretty well satisfied that I've done a comprehensive search.

Earlier, you mentioned that doctors have to help their patients be wary of information they find on the Web. That really goes for all of us. How would you compare medical information on the Web to what we can get from a source like MEDLINE?

The fact that MEDLINE is now available to consumers is a good thing. Compared with much of the information that's out there, the articles in MEDLINE go through a peer review process. That doesn't mean that you should automatically do whatever MEDLINE tells you to do, but at least you have peer review on your side.

As you know, just because it's on the Web doesn't mean it's true. There's a wonderful anecdote about the "exploding head syndrome" [165]. It's written up as a true case, so you read it and think, "Oh, my gosh, I wonder if this really happened. Oh my." It sounds just like a real case reported in very clinical terms, but it's a total hoax—a spoof to show how anything can be couched in language that will make it seem real, when in fact there's no truth to it at all.

As information professionals, we need to remind people about healthy skepticism. When our students make a statement, we always ask, "What evidence is there for that? Where did you find that? Quote your source. What year was that published in?" It's our role to remind people that not everything is of equal value, not everything is as reliable as it may seem, and a healthy dose of skepticism is still a very good way to approach any information, whether Web-, book-, or online-journal-based.

What databases do you use besides MEDLINE?

HealthSTAR [93], CINAHL [127] (Cumulative Index to Nursing and Allied Health), and Cochrane Collaboration [128]. HealthSTAR focuses on the clinical outcomes and the effectiveness of practice, as well as the non-clinical aspects of healthcare delivery, such as administration, economics, planning, and policy. The Cochrane

Collaboration is a voluntary effort to bring together tools to help get at the best evidence-based medicine resources. It's an international network of healthcare professionals who review the literature and write appraisals of each article, including whether it does or does not answer a particular clinical question. There are headquarters all over the world, including McMaster in Canada, groups in England and Japan, and in the United States as well.

I occasionally use EMBASE [131], though not in quite awhile. The cost is rather prohibitive, but it certainly is a good resource. When someone is doing comprehensive kinds of writing, we will do an EMBASE search for them. It includes more European journals and good early drug research.

Would you use any Web-based resources?

We use a set of Web pages called HealthWeb [4], which was originally created by a group of midwestern medical school libraries. We divvied up the various specialty areas; each medical library took on certain disciplines and made a point of looking at the Web in those specialty areas. We agreed on a format, reviewed all kinds of Web sites, and catalogued them.

HealthWeb is a series of annotated and reviewed links. We've actually looked at each of those sites and made a decision that, yes, this is good enough to include. The links are also updated on a regular basis; we review them regularly. In addition, as librarians, we show our pages to active professionals in the discipline and ask, "What do you think? Have we left anything out? Is this useful?"

One nice thing about HealthWeb is that it is not only annotated and reviewed, but it is also a uniform platform with the same look and feel across the board. We've won awards and the press has said some nice things about us.

If we went to HealthWeb, what would we find?

I'm responsible for Health Informatics. There's a general first page. Then there are guides to Health Informatics resources, clinical and educational resources, academic institutions and research programs, organizations, electronic publications, electronic communications, conferences and events, career opportunities, and finally, miscellaneous resources. This is a uniform format across all disciplines.

Beyond HealthWeb, how do you decide where to send physicians for information on the Web?

My criteria are, first, the reliability and authority of the site and, secondly, whether that site would provide a jumping-off point. One of my favorites is Medical Matrix [8]. Medical Matrix is arranged by specialty and is also keyword-searchable. What I like about it is that it ranks sites like movie reviews, with a five-star system. The site is governed by an editorial board, so you know who's selecting these sites, and the lists are annotated and updated very frequently. It's very well put-together, probably one of my all-time favorites. Other favorites include: PubMed, of course; MedHunt [7]; Medical World Search [9]; Healthfinder [3] (consumer information); DrKoop.com [18] (consumer information); 1stHeadlines-Health [33]; MedWeb [11], from Emory University Health Sciences Center Library; The Virtual Hospital [14]; and the American College of Physicians-American Society for Internal Medicine (ACP-ASIM) home page for internists [71].

Do you keep your sites organized?

Sort of. I rely on my bookmarks. I've got my search engines and then my evidence-based medicine sites grouped together. I teach an Informatics curriculum, so I like to see what other schools are doing in informatics. There are informatics curriculum servers in Medical Informatics, Healthcare Telematics and Telemedicine, and so on. Anything I haven't had a chance to organize is at the very end; I file them about once a month. I also back up my bookmarks, because I lost my whole bookmarks file once, and it was just devastating.

Fran, since you often have to tell others about good sites, how do you keep up with new sources yourself?

It's challenging. Mainly through word of mouth, in discussion groups. Medical librarians have their own discussion group, MEDLIB-L [174]. So does the Association of Academic Health Sciences Library Directors [74]. If one of us hears something, we pass it along. When I get something through a mailing list, I pass it on to the staff here. It all comes back to networking, talking to other people and saying, "Oh, that sounds good," when you're told of a new source. It's about being open and being someone that other people tell things to. That means being open to new and different things so that you radiate that interest.

With the wealth of information available now, what do you think is missing?

What's missing is timely information at the point of care. If I were a clinician talking to my patient in an inpatient situation, I should be able to use a palmtop or laptop or whatever to access some information service, input my question, and get an answer in real time. That's what's missing. I can see the hospital out my window, with the clinician at the patient's bedside, and I'm over here with all this information.

Right now, physicians can get the same information that I can, but they may not know how to do it quickly and efficiently. What I hope is to teach them how to become better self-directed learners, and then make it easier for them to do their own literature searches.

Is there any final point you want to make?

It's important to keep focused on our function as information professionals, as opposed to the process or the technology. Sometimes we get caught up in the process, or a particular technology. But the important thing is how you evaluate information, no matter what format it's in. Sure, evaluating the Web is different from evaluating a journal article, but there are common things that you look for: Who's the authority, is an author identified, when was it last updated, is it backed by an organization, what are the credentials of the person putting it forth?

Our function is to collect, organize, disseminate, and facilitate the use of information and to teach others how to do that.

Super Searcher Power Tips

➤ On teaching evidence-based medicine to medical students

The key to finding clinical information is to first formulate your question. This question has four parts: Who is the patient, what is the intervention, what are you comparing it to, and what outcomes are you looking for?

➤ On maintaining a healthy skepticism

When our students make a statement, we always ask, "What evidence is there for that? Where did you find that? Quote your source. What year was that published in?" Not everything is of equal value, not everything is as reliable as it may seem, and a healthy dose of skepticism is still a very good way to approach any information, whether Web-, book-, or online-journal-based.

➤ On starting a Web search for medical information

HealthWeb is a series of annotated and reviewed links. They're updated on a regular basis. We show them to active professionals and ask, "What do you think? Have we left anything out? Is this useful?"

➤ On the importance of networking to keep up with sources

Networking is about being open and being someone that other people tell things to. That means being open to new and different things so that you radiate that interest.

➤ On evaluating information

Sure, evaluating the Web is different from evaluating a journal article, but there are common things that you look for: Who's the authority, is there an author identified, when was it last updated, is it backed by an organization, what are the credentials of the person putting this forth?

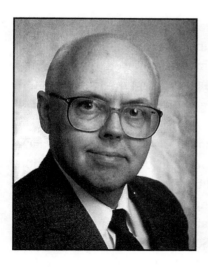

Thomas Emmett

Doctor Turned Librarian

Thomas Emmett, M.D., M.L.S., is the Reference Systems Coordinator for the Ruth Lilly Medical Library at Indiana University in Indianapolis, and Adjunct Professor of Knowledge Informatics at the Indiana University School of Medicine in Indianapolis.

temmett@iupui.edu

Tom, your background is different from most medical librarians. Having gotten an M.D. first, I imagine you have a closer feel for the clinician's needs. How did you end up on the librarian side?

I followed the traditional pathway into medicine with undergraduate and medical degrees from the University of Iowa. Early on, I developed a very strong interest in information organization. During my early residency years here at Indiana University, I began to create a card file, indexing articles with terms that I initially just picked out of the air. Along the way, I realized that it was important to have some organization to these terms. It became a very interesting hobby for me. I ended up creating about 200 typed pages of my own "MeSH vocabulary" with all the hierarchical relationships and cross-references that I had found to be useful.

After 13 years of practice, I was interested in looking at other avenues to further my career, and to deviate a bit from the constraints of managed care medicine. I was very naive with regard to the world of library science and had no idea what discipline paralleled my interests. Once "information science" became a part of traditional library programs, the light went on and I knew where I wanted to head. From 1992 to1994, I pursued a master's degree in library science at the Indiana University School of Library and Information Science.

I felt it was very important not to discard my medical background and figured that I would probably be in a unique position, once I understood the basics of library science, to be able to pass this expertise along in a teaching mode to students, residents, and other healthcare professionals. I was fortunate to have been offered a position here at the IU School of Medicine Library (Ruth Lilly Medical Library), and I've been here ever since.

So medical librarianship is a refuge from managed care?

I guess that's right. It's really an interesting field, and it's a refuge from HMOs, but it also allows me to get into medical education more than I was able to in the past. That's the ultimate challenge—once you've got a knowledge base, you try to pass it on to other people. Medical librarianship allows me to do that very effectively.

Who are your clients now?

Here at the School of Medicine, we have a built-in clientele in the faculty, staff, and students of the IU Schools of Nursing, Medicine, and Allied Health. Our mission is to serve primarily these groups of people. The vast majority of my online searches concern clinical medicine and nursing topics as applied to direct patient care and research. I also do a small number of searches for consumers, and we get a few personal injury attorney requests for information and guidelines on specific types of injuries. We also serve non-IU physicians and other health professionals throughout the state.

Certainly, my medical background has been a tremendous asset in developing strategies and in quality filtering.

Can you expand on that?

I can understand the client's request a lot better. When I walk away, I know what they want; I don't struggle with the medical terminology. Sometimes I may not totally understand it, but I know what to ask in order to clarify. My experience helps me understand the narrower concepts they may want to include or exclude, which is an advantage over a medical librarian who doesn't have the extensive subject background.

When you get a reference question, where do you go first?

Probably 75 to 80 percent of my searches are done in MED-LINE [96, see Appendix A] and CINAHL [127]. Depending on the topic and the patron's wishes, I'll expand to include a number of other databases. For basic science, I add BIOSIS [123]. For drug-related questions, I'll consider searching EMBASE [131], International Pharmaceutical Abstracts [138], and AIDSDRUGS [82], but most definitely will search Micromedex [167].

Micromedex is invaluable for current, well-referenced drug information. I believe it's almost exclusively written by PharmDs. Its REPRORISK [29] files are particularly useful for questions about drug use during pregnancy.

For cancer and AIDS-related questions, I'll check CANCERLIT [83] and AIDSLINE [82] for meeting abstracts. From experience, I've found that the meeting abstracts are almost always the only non-MEDLINE records in those two files. Then I'll check CancerNet [84] for state-of-the-art monographs.

Clinical trials information is best found on PDQ [111] for cancer, AIDSTRIALS [82] for AIDS, and Web sources like CenterWatch.com [126] for other disease categories.

Where there's a clear psychological component, like irritable bowel syndrome or behavioral interventions in cancer screening, searching PsycINFO [146] is a must. Sometimes I'll even check ERIC [132], particularly if there's an educational aspect to the question, like academic achievement in seizure patients.

What about very basic research, like genetics?

Here at IU, the genetics sequencing databases are primarily searched by researchers themselves, although one of my colleagues is developing the expertise to provide assistance when needed. For more general information on genetic diseases, the OMIM [109] (Online Mendelian Inheritance in Man) database on the Web is extremely complete. Those are certainly not for the consumer, though; the monographs are geared toward the genetics researcher. If we need more consumer-friendly information, the print *Birth Defects Encyclopedia* [177] is also valuable.

You've touched on consumer questions. Where else would you go to help out the non-professional?

At the Lilly Library we don't maintain a large consumer collection, so I depend heavily on the Web. There are a number of high-quality sites, but I like to check MEDLINEplus [97] first, because of its wide range of topics and its links to government and professional sites that aren't cluttered with advertising. Familydoctor.org [20] from the American Academy of Family Physicians is also a good site, but it covers fewer topics. I've bookmarked a number of commercial and educational sites, but I don't really favor them in any particular order—Mayo Clinic Health Oasis [23], ThriveOnline [31], Healthfinder [3], HealthWeb [4]. Sometimes I'll use a general search engine like HotBot [150] or AltaVista [149], and just see what I get, but then I have to do some heavy quality filtering. I feel I'm able to tell quickly where the information's coming from and whether it's worthwhile.

Let's go back to searching for medical professionals. What do you need to know before you can start your search?

If I'm dealing with a medical topic, I often have a general idea about how much is out there. I use that as a basis for deciding what specific additional information I need. It's very important to know what the patron is going to do with the information: Is he writing a case report? A systematic review? Giving a presentation to an audience of his peers? To a group of medical students? Is the information for direct patient care, or just keeping up in one's research area?

Asking how much the patron expects to find, or how much he's willing to read, is also important. This is especially helpful for patient-care questions; quite often, if an answer can be found in a few current articles, nothing else is needed.

What about those comprehensive questions, where the requestor begins with "I want everything on ..."?

Then I want to know if cost is a factor and whether they are really prepared to pay for and read through 500 or 1,000 records. In an academic setting, cost often *is* a factor, and when I bring that up, the nature of the request can change completely; the requestor becomes more serious about what they actually want. I've found that, when a patron really *does* want a comprehensive search, they are often knowledgeable about the specific databases they want to include, and that is certainly important for me to know.

If the search doesn't really have to be comprehensive, I try to negotiate some reasonable limits to apply. Is it okay to limit to human and English-language studies? Can I exclude letters to the editor? Can I limit to local holdings? Can I limit to only the last one or two years? I try to make sure I am completely clear on what the requestor wants before I waste any time going down the wrong path.

Since you rely heavily on MEDLINE, how about walking me through the search process?

We use Ovid [158], so I'll be referring to Ovid's features. But when setting up MEDLINE strategies, I follow a fairly standard procedure that most searchers probably follow. I first track down all relevant subject headings in each of my concept groups by using, in order, Ovid's mapping feature, the permuted index, and, finally, title words to locate "on target" articles. I then check the indexing of those articles for additional headings. If title words continue to retrieve useful articles even after I've added all relevant headings to the strategy, I'll retain them as search terms.

Depending on the amount of retrieval and the level of comprehensiveness required, I'll add text words. You have to remember the need to use truncation, for example, to pick up possessives like "Alzheimer's." You have to account for spelling variations—for example, American versus British—and hyphenation variants. It always amazes me; if it is at all possible to divide a single word into two by using a space or a hyphen, then someone will do it in a MEDLINE record. And both variants have to be included in the search strategy.

I've constructed a number of hedges over the years to help me when searching for certain recurring topics, and I try to keep those close at hand so as not to waste time recreating them.

What kinds of hedges are those?

Some examples are limiting to children, the elderly, or pregnant patients—including both pregnancy and pregnancy complications. For children, there are some good journal words to consider, like "child" or "pediatric," that would immediately limit to this age group. For nutritional topics like "nutritional aspects of (a specific disease)," there are many very closely related headings. The ones that begin with the word "dietary"—for example, dietary fats or dietary proteins—are easy to overlook because they are not part of the main nutrition trees.

Do you ever use PubMed [112]?

Yes, I use PubMed quite often for updating my Ovid searches with the most current MEDLINE and PreMEDLINE records. I'll occasionally use PubMed as a cross-check for the strategies I create in Ovid MEDLINE, particularly on searches with a very low yield. PubMed's default strategies and the "Related Records" algorithm use text words very liberally, even when identical subject headings are available. That makes it a quick way to check for missed relevant records that might allow me to fine-tune my strategy.

There are two downsides to using these built-in PubMed search modes. First, retrieval is often low-recall, meaning that related relevant headings are not picked up; secondly, it's often low-precision, as when searching "all fields" for every concept leads to a lot of false drops.

One important point to remember when searching PubMed for PreMEDLINE records is to include text words in all your concept groups. Since these most current records haven't been indexed yet, searching with MeSH terms alone will miss them. PubMed is still very cumbersome for setting up strategies from scratch, but I'm hoping that future enhancements will make this easier.

Besides its currency, one nice feature about PubMed is the ability to set up links on a Web page that will automatically run search strategies in PubMed. I can set up these links for my current awareness customers, direct them to the Web page where they're located, and let them run their updates anytime they wish. Theoretically, these links can also be sent via email using a client like Microsoft Outlook, but I haven't been able to get the long URLs to wrap correctly in the body of the message.

With your medical background, do your requestors expect you to preview and filter the results before you send them?

The degree of filtering I do, beyond applying limits, varies depending on what the patron expects. Generally, the tolerance for irrelevant records is pretty low, so I do some fairly serious filtering, particularly if I'm familiar with the subject. If a faculty member is considering writing a case report, and nothing in the literature directly matches his parameters, I'll expand the search to look for the reports that match most closely. Maybe a particular drug hasn't been shown to cause a specific side effect, but another one in its class has. Of course, when I expand the search like this, I have to be sure to explain in detail what I've done, so the patron doesn't think I misunderstood the question.

Evidence-based medicine (EBM) is being taught a lot at medical schools. What's the thrust behind this movement?

Evidence-based medicine has really come to the fore in medical education with its premise that therapeutic interventions should be tested in controlled clinical trials or other appropriate study types in order to prove their value. This means a strong emphasis on efficient searching of newer evidence-based databases and on applying evidence-based limits to older databases like MEDLINE.

The EBM movement has dramatically increased our medical library's involvement in the curriculum at all levels. We've begun to demonstrate these search techniques in Internal Medicine Morning Report, a teaching conference generally run by the chief medicine resident, where an interesting patient case is presented. Our role is to help a resident conduct a MEDLINE search on a topic related to the case, demonstrating how to incorporate evidence-based research into patient care.

But I almost never use the strategies developed for evidence-based searching when I perform a MEDLINE search for a faculty member. They're almost exclusively tools to be taught to future practitioners and used in patient-care situations for quickly narrowing output to the most clinically relevant material. It would be a rare researcher who requested, for example, that we limit a subject search exclusively to randomized, controlled trials.

When you do conduct EBM searches, what's your process?

I always start with MEDLINE for applying evidence-based hedges, because most of the EBM research has been done in this database. The ground-breaking study by Haynes et al. [183] established eight strategies for limiting to the evidence-based literature in the areas of etiology, prognosis, diagnosis, and therapy. Back in 1991, these strategies were found to be the most sensitive and specific when tested against records from 10 journals. However, I feel it's important to include additional terms, particularly publication types for therapy articles, such as "controlled clinical trial" and "randomized controlled trial." This gives you a more comprehensive retrieval and takes advantage of better indexing by the National Library of Medicine since that time.

Ann McKibbon included a number of expanded strategies in her book, *PDQ: Evidence-Based Principles and Practice* [185]. I highly recommend this book to anyone involved in teaching evidence-based searching.

Where else might you find EBM literature?

The Cochrane Controlled Trials Register [128] is an important alternative to MEDLINE for locating controlled clinical trials. This is one of four databases produced by the Cochrane Collaboration as part of the Cochrane Library, which is now on the Web. There's a working arrangement between the Cochrane Centers and the NLM to locate and properly tag all controlled clinical trials in MEDLINE. So there's some significant overlap between these two databases. However, I still search both to maximize my retrieval.

For locating systematic reviews, I like to first search the Cochrane Database of Systematic Reviews [128] and then, for non-Cochrane reviews, DARE [130], the Database of Abstracts of Reviews of Effectiveness. MEDLINE doesn't do as good a job of indexing systematic reviews, particularly those that aren't identified as meta-analyses, so you need a complex hedge to isolate them.

Another strategy I like to use for locating evidence-based studies is the "limit to EBM reviews" feature of Ovid MEDLINE. This lets me take advantage of MeSH indexing in constructing a strategy, which I can then limit to only those articles that have been included in a Cochrane systematic review or reviewed for inclusion in *ACP Journal Club* [42] or *Evidence-Based Medicine* [52]. Then I can link directly to these reviews.

Do you ever search full text?

Rarely—not unless the concepts are highly specific, and I've come up empty in the bibliographic files. There are some interesting circumstances, however, in which full-text searching can be very rewarding. If you want to identify cases where the patient had a constellation of historical or physical findings—say, fever, chest pain, and pleural effusion—then entering these terms into a full-text database might pick up very useful discussions about the differential diagnosis.

Another example, which occurred recently, was a patron looking for articles containing decision trees or decision models. He wasn't interested in articles that were *about* these subjects, unless the article also contained the actual tree or model. Neither the "decision trees" heading nor the abstracts eliminated false drops. So, the most precise strategy seemed to be to go into the full-text collections available on Ovid, and search the caption text under the graphics for "decision adj3 (tree: or model:)." This yielded a much more useful set of records that couldn't have been retrieved without full-text searching.

It's always a fun challenge to help court reporters and transcriptionists figure out the garbled words a doctor is saying. Often, I don't have any idea either, but full-text or MEDLINE searching frequently turns up the answer. MEDLINE is also a great spell checker, particularly when a patron wants to know whether a word is typically hyphenated or not; I can see how many times in titles and abstracts it is and isn't.

Speaking of full text, do you ever use textbooks online?

Electronic textbooks are helpful when I'm searching for a factual piece of information that's no longer the subject of medical debate or research. I prefer the multi-work collections of STAT!Ref

[41], which includes more than 30 texts, and MD Consult [6], with more than 35 texts, to the single-text sites like Harrison's Online [39] and Scientific American Medicine Online [66], because you can accomplish more with a single strategy. STAT!Ref has a very sophisticated search system that allows searching across the full text of all its references using proximity operators ADJ or NEAR/x. The matching words in each retrieved text are highlighted.

By contrast, MD Consult only searches the back-of-the-book indexes of each text, so the strategies have to be much more general. Then again, MD Consult has chosen to target the physician searcher almost exclusively, and so intentionally decided against full-text searching and its greater possibility for irrelevant retrieval. As a more experienced searcher, though, I find this very unsatisfactory when I'm looking for a specific fact.

I generally use other Web-based texts less often, but several good ones are freely available, like the Iowa Family Practice Handbook [40] and the emergency medicine text at emedicine.com [38].

Which kinds of searches do you enjoy most?

There are several that I find rewarding. I really enjoy searching the literature for case reports of rare medical conditions for physicians who are considering writing a case report themselves. Recently, I had one dealing with hepatic failure caused by an overdose of the anti-migraine drug sumatriptan. When I found nothing, I broadened the search to include all liver diseases and all triptan drugs, just to see what the closest association might be. This tactic wouldn't be helpful, of course, if there were a lot of results, but it's highly informative when there are very little.

I also feel a great sense of accomplishment whenever I can use the citation indexes to verify older or difficult citations. These are incredible tools that often eliminate the need to manually search the old *Index Medicus* volumes. Unfortunately, they're very expensive and might not be practical for frequent use without an institutional licensing agreement.

Could you explore that a bit more for me? When would you need to use a citation index, and how would you use it?

Someone might walk up with a page from a book chapter or a meeting abstract and want to know where it came from. If you're lucky enough to have an author name and a page number, then a cited reference search will often provide the answer. This also works well for identifying other publication types, like dissertations, which are less likely to be indexed in the more traditional databases. Science Citation Index [140] and its Web-based counterpart, ISI's Web of Science [140], are the principal tools used for this kind of searching.

Citation indexes are also valuable for providing support to people seeking tenure. If they give us a complete bibliography of their publications, then we can tell them how many times each has been cited.

The citation databases are incredible for verifying citations from further back in the literature, because the index isn't limited by years. A lot of retired physicians really latch onto the history of medicine-type topics; they're interested in the older literature, and they can trace citations back with it. Even if the index only covers articles published in the last 10 years, you can still verify a citation from 1955; all it requires is that somebody within the last 10 years has cited that same work.

From the older literature to the new, how do you keep up with all the changes and new information resources, much less the changes that are happening in medicine itself?

I don't spend as much time keeping up as I would like, but I guess everyone has that problem. I'm trying to maintain my expertise in both internal medicine and library science, so I'm faced with an impossible task.

The sources that I try to review regularly for new database information are the *NLM Technical Bulletin* [62], the *JAMA NetSight* [5] series of articles which identify the "best" Web sites in a specialty, the American College of Physicians' Web Sites for Internists [15], and *Medicine on the Net* [59]. Within our library, we also circulate several periodicals like *EContent* [51] and *Searcher* [68], from which I extract the medically-related information. I also subscribe to *Information Today* [56], which occasionally focuses on medical database searching. The only electronic mailing list to which I belong is MEDLIB-L [174], but this is often a good source of information for online searchers, particularly Peg Allen's valuable CINAHL contributions.

If you could have any kind of resource or change anything about searching, what would that be? What would make your work easier?

The major "pie-in-the-sky" request I would make—that would actually be doable—would be for the National Library of Medicine to make PubMed as fully functional as ELHILL was and to approach Ovid's capabilities as much as possible. This would include making all fields available for searching that had been available in ELHILL, providing true adjacency searching, and allowing unlimited truncation.

I'm annoyed that PubMed didn't retain the entry month or date-of-entry fields that correspond to the monthly or weekly updates supplied by vendors like Ovid. As a result, there is no way to cleanly segregate the most current records .in PubMed from those already retrieved in Ovid, and manual scanning is required to avoid duplicates.

Real "pie-in-the-sky" changes—that will *never* happen—would be for EMBASE to be just as inexpensive to search as MEDLINE or, ideally, for the two databases to combine with a thesaurus that incorporates the best features of both. An interim dream would be an easier way to exclude MEDLINE records from EMBASE.

My final wishes are for faster, near-instantaneous, Web-based searching and the availability of all full text in Adobe PDF format.

Super Searcher Power Tips

➤ On using text words in searches

You have to remember the need to use truncation, for example, to pick up possessives like "Alzheimer's." You have to account for spelling variations—for example, American versus British—and hyphenation variants. It always amazes me; if it is at all possible to divide a single word into two by using a space or a hyphen, then someone will do it in a MEDLINE record. And both variants have to be included in the search strategy.

➤ On using PubMed as a professional searcher

I'll occasionally use PubMed as a cross-check for the strategies I create in Ovid MEDLINE, particularly on searches with a very low yield. PubMed's default strategies and the "Related Records" algorithm use textwords very liberally, even when identical subject headings are available. That makes it a quick way to check for missed relevant records that might allow me to fine-tune my strategy.

➤ On using PubMed for current awareness

Besides its currency, one feature about PubMed that I really like is the ability to set up links on a Web page that will automatically run search strategies in PubMed. I can set up these links for my current awareness customers, direct them to the Web page where they're located, and let them run their updates anytime they wish.

➤ On the limitations of evidence-based medicine

I almost never use the strategies developed for evidence-based searching when I perform a MEDLINE search for a faculty member. They're almost exclusively tools to be taught to future practitioners and used in patient-care situations for quickly narrowing output to the most clinically relevant material. It would be a rare researcher who requested, for example, that we limit a subject search exclusively to randomized, controlled trials.

➤ On using electronic textbooks

Electronic textbooks are helpful when I'm searching for a factual piece of information that's no longer the subject of medical debate or research. I prefer the multi-work collections of STAT!Ref and MD Consult to the single-text sites like Harrison's Online and Scientific American Medicine Online, because you can accomplish more with a single strategy.

➤ On using citation indexes

One way is to put in the name of the first author of a particular article and find out who cited that article; it's a way to bring out the more current literature that has cited an article that you've initially identified. The citation databases are incredible for verifying citations from further back in the literature, because the index isn't limited by years.

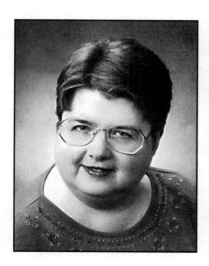

Margaret (Peg) Allen

Serving Allied Health

Peg Allen, M.L.S., A.H.I.P., is an independent library consultant specializing in public and allied health information. She is based in Stratford, Wisconsin.

pegallen@tznet.com

Peg, your signature line is extensive. It includes M.L.S., A.H.I.P., library information consultant, resource librarian consultant for CINAHL Information Systems, Inc., and library consultant for Northern Wisconsin Area Health Education Center, Inc. What's your background and how did you come to wear all those hats?

My goal in library school was not to get too focused on anything in particular because I wasn't sure what I wanted to do, so I took a wide variety of classes. My first job out of library school was in a hospital library where I was the first professional librarian. I was hired to serve the entire hospital staff, not just the physicians, which was a new concept for this hospital. After a few years, I merged that library with the nursing library, which made it a lot easier to serve the nursing staff as well as the students and faculty of the diploma and B.S.N. nursing schools there.

Then we moved to northern Wisconsin, and I got a nursing school library job at St. Joseph's Hospital School of Nursing in

Marshfield. Eventually, the library moved into the main hospital and merged with the patient library. We had a lot of challenges keeping the school going, as our nursing program evolved from a diploma school to a four-year program. The National League for Nursing accreditation requirements for faculty kept going up, so I was helping faculty get their master's degrees. Due to accreditation requirements, I became part of the nursing school faculty and participated in all their meetings. I was there for 15 years. The school closed in 1988, but it was replaced by a satellite program of the University of Wisconsin–Eau Claire.

At the same time, in the mid-'80s, I started teaching the Medical Library Association Continuing Education (MLACE) course in Nursing Information Access. It's an eight-hour course for librarians. A fair amount of the course is about the nursing profession and how it's different from other health professions— you know, really getting at their information needs, what their work environment is, trying to see things from their point of view. I am a strong believer in getting to know your clients and their needs before you go out trying to find information for them.

How do the research needs of a nursing or allied health professional differ from those of a physician?

Number one, nursing has a professional identity crisis, so they have tried over the years to develop their own theoretical foundation in something other than the biomedical model as a basis for their practice. They consider other aspects of human health or, as they say, they treat the human response to health and illness. There is a greater emphasis on psychosocial resources. Secondly, their accreditation criteria place a much greater emphasis on teaching techniques and educational soundness than I think medical school accreditation does. All this means that you have to have access to the purely medical literature, plus the nursing literature, plus psychosocial resources and education literature. In a nutshell, nurses need a much broader range of subject material.

How did the CINAHL [127, see Appendix A] database develop?

CINAHL is the Cumulative Index to Nursing and Allied Health Literature, which started in hard copy as a nursing index in the late 1950s. It went electronic in 1983. From the beginning, it was multi-format. It's not a journal article database, although that's what most people seem to believe. It also covers books, audiovisuals, software, government documents, and now Web sites.

Most of the database is citation format, but government documents—anything that's in the public domain—are in full text. They also have copyright permission from many of the state nursing journals to include those articles in full text. The CINAHL database has a field for Web site URLs, so that if an article discusses Web sites in depth, the URLs are included. The searcher doesn't even have to go to the article itself to get the Web references. CINAHL also lists all the cited references for cooperating journals, so there's a whole field of bibliographies you can search. Quite a different database.

The CINAHL Web site indexing is my role, believe it or not. When we started including Web sites, it would have been possible to keep up with all the nursing and allied health sites. Now, I don't think I'll ever catch up, especially as we try to include all the consumer health Web sites as well. The Web site descriptions are also available on the CINAHL Web site as the CINAHL*sources* link index.

Has your experience with indexing colored your approach to searching?

Yes. I worked for awhile as editor of International Nursing Index [137] (INI), where the journal indexing represents the nursing information in HealthSTAR [93] and MEDLINE [96]. INI also includes additional print-only sections such as a Nursing

Thesaurus guide to MeSH, nursing books, dissertations, and statistics sources. I learned that they receive absolutely no income from the National Library of Medicine [103] for producing the International Nursing Index, nor does the American Hospital Association [73] for HealthSTAR, the Health Planning and Administration Index. The American Dental Association [72] receives absolutely no income for the indexing they do that goes into MEDLINE and the Index to Dental Literature [136]. As a result, new titles are not being added to these databases as fast as they might be with a product like CINAHL, which isn't dependent on NLM [103] for income. Indexing is expensive, as you might imagine.

So, the associations are practically volunteering to do the indexing?

Yes, and in return they would get clean copy for their own index and revenue from the print versions that they produced. When the National Library of Medicine announced free access to the world in 1997, the bottom of the print market suddenly dropped out. All of these organizations are struggling with how they can continue to support this indexing activity for the professions they serve.

So, all those wonderful high-quality indexes that we've come to rely on are not necessarily growing or adding new publications. What are our options for getting at the missing material?

Unfortunately, with free MEDLINE, it's hard to convince people that you have to pay for a good search interface, or that you have to pay for other databases. It may not matter to the average clinician, but the pure researcher needs to search a lot of different sources and have access to a top-notch search engine. You have to search the commercial databases too, if you're going to do a thorough search. If I were serving medicine, I would be using

EMBASE [131] a lot more. I don't think there's any excuse, if you're dealing with nursing and allied health, for not using CINAHL.

Besides MEDLINE, what would you add to CINAHL when you do an allied health search?

This is an amazing thing. A few years ago, I began some research that took the Brandon Hill [184] list of books and journals for allied health, one of the three standard core lists for medical libraries, and looked at where most of the titles were indexed. This was presented at MLA [77] in 1993, as "The Core of the Bibliographic Apple" [178]. It varied from field to field, but I discovered that some allied health fields, like music therapy and education, are better covered in PsycLIT [146]. EMBASE picked up quite a few for physical therapy, ERIC [132] for language and speech pathology, and for any service provided by the schools. A lot of our health services today are provided in schools; that's where the kids are.

The Nursing and Allied Health Resources Section (NAHRS) of the Medical Library Association continued research in this area, using bibliometric analysis of the citations for core journals in selected allied health disciplines, and is publishing results as the research is completed. Barbara Schloman, chair of this task force, was invited to speak to NLM's Literature Selection and Review Committee about this research, and both CINAHL and MEDLINE coverage of allied health journals has increased.

It sounds like you can't always tell where you're going to find the information.

You have to search multiple databases if you really want to be comprehensive. It's not just MEDLINE. MEDLINE is adding allied health fields more slowly because they're newer fields. The journal selection criteria for *Index Medicus* are very stringent. They're looking for research literature. A lot of the allied health fields are just beginning to mature and develop their own research literature, so the journals don't get picked up as quickly in MEDLINE via the *Index Medicus* route. I have been told that whether a health sciences journal is indexed in MEDLINE or not is a make-or-break factor, unfortunately, in terms of its commercial success.

I'd like you to put on your other hat for a little while. What is the Northern Wisconsin Area Health Education Center?

The Area Health Education Centers (AHEC) in the United States are part of a federal program that provides start-up funding for states to help increase the supply of health professionals and improve healthcare in underserved communities. Several states now have AHEC programs, mostly funded with state revenues, grants, and income from services. The AHECs are involved in everything from supporting medical student rotations in rural and inner-city communities, to sponsoring week-long cultural diversity immersion experiences and, in many parts of the country, providing library services for rural areas. Northern Wisconsin Area Health Education Center [119] (NAHEC) serves the northern 38 counties in Wisconsin, which are primarily rural. We also have Native American partners and organizations serving the Hmong people from southeast Asia, as well as some that serve migrant workers. Recently, I started working with the Southwest Wisconsin AHEC (SWAHEC) to develop library/information programs for its region.

What kind of research services do you provide for them?

In this case, I'm my own customer. I do grant writing and program development and do my own searches for the grants. For these, I need to know about community characteristics and population health problems, which you can usually get from the individual state Department of Health Web sites. A lot of the research involves working with the partners and determining their library/health information needs using surveys and focus groups. In rural Wisconsin, our partners include healthcare organizations such as clinics, hospitals, and county health departments, as well as small colleges and technical schools.

In our consumer health projects, we will also be working with schools, public libraries, and departments of aging. Then you need background literature to support how programs can make a difference, which means looking into the medical education, informatics, and nursing and allied health education literature for what might have been successful elsewhere. Unfortunately, most library outreach projects are not very well documented. A lot of these projects are presented at conferences, such as national AHEC workshops and MLA, and lost. Many final reports are submitted to the funding agencies, but personnel are so busy trying to meet needs, they simply don't have the time to write scholarly articles for peer-reviewed journals. Also, many librarians move on when the grant funding ends.

Do you use the Internet a lot in your research?

Definitely, what with the health statistics Web sites, access to Ovid [158] full-text databases because of the Wisconsin AHEC partnership with the University of Wisconsin–Madison Medical School, and Internet access to full-text databases from our Wisconsin BadgerLink [116] project. BadgerLink is a state-funded initiative, which gives all Wisconsin citizens and students access to EBSCO [162] databases—including three that focus on health information—plus large academic, public, and school library collections.

We also have access to a collection of national and Wisconsin newspapers from Bell & Howell's ProQuest [169] service. The indexing isn't as good as it is in MEDLINE and CINAHL, though. That gets to be more and more of a problem as we move more and more toward the Web. I am a very strong believer in controlled vocabulary, combined with text word; you can't get it all from text-word searching.

What do you lose with text-word searching?

You lose all the synonyms. For example, someone was looking for experiences precepting nursing students and new nurses. If that person didn't also look under "mentorship" or "mentoring," he or she would miss an awful lot of the literature. However, a controlled vocabulary term will get you to the whole concept, regardless of how it's described.

The other thing we have in medicine, which we don't always seem to appreciate, is the fact that the controlled vocabularies for both CINAHL and MEDLINE are in tree structures. You can go up and down the tree; if you're not getting enough with the term you've picked, you can go broader, or you can explode headings to get the narrower headings from underneath.

Most good searchers prefer to choose their own search method, depending on the question. Unfortunately, the Web-based systems from NLM explode automatically, whether you want them to or not, so you end up losing precision. If you need to go broader, you have to do a lot of truncated searches and be very good with synonyms, or you lose some hits.

At the same time, you get too much if you rely on text-word searching, because you get a lot of false drops. Many of the words used in medicine, like "clinical" or "case management," show up again and again. In fact, "case management" is a terrible subject to search; if you just search on that phrase, you get management of a particular case, which is something different altogether.

If you're trying to be comprehensive, you have to add text words. Generally, though, if I'm getting more than enough information, I will rely on subject headings alone.

What about a new field, where the indexing might not have caught up to the topic?

Then you need to use text-word searching. Again, NLM is very slow to adopt new terminology. I'm sure you've heard of a medical assistant? "Medical assistant" is not a MeSH term; "physician assistant" is. MeSH vocabulary is extremely biomedical. It doesn't really take into account the full range of allied health professions. It is impossible to do a precise search on the subject of medical assistants in HealthSTAR or MEDLINE on the NLM systems today.

One thing I learned as editor of the International Nursing Index is that many database producers are more likely to listen to suggestions for new terms from searchers than they are from their own indexers. That, of course, increases the time it takes for new vocabulary to get in. Fortunately, this is not true for CINAHL!

Peg, I've noticed on MEDLIB-L [174] that you always know the answer to "Where do I find this?" You tell them how to look for it and the caveats about relying on the information when they find it.

CINAHL recruited me because they liked that online advice. I'm doing customer service by providing search help online. I do this for nursing and other health professional mailing lists, too. A good source for nursing lists is the "Mailing Lists" section of Nursing & Health Care Resources on the Net [13].

People who haven't had access to any information at all are overwhelmed with what's out there for free. This is particularly true for health professionals at our rural partner sites. When we teach, we talk a lot about evaluating what they find. We teach them to use the free databases they have access to and to use metasites on the Internet. I'm a firm believer in subject directories or meta-sites. We de-emphasize using the major search engines, because they're just going to get too much information back.

Any particular consumer sites you send them to?

I like HealthWeb [4], which is a set of Web sites with a unified look and feel that's produced by a number of libraries. Each one takes a discipline within medicine and builds the Web site in a compatible format. If I'm trying to find sites in a particular field, I pay attention to the Hardin MD [2] directory from the University of Iowa, which consists of lists of subject directories and evaluations of their hits. For consumers, the health topics in MEDLINE*plus* [97] are getting to be quite good, as are the health topics in Healthfinder [3] from the government.

NOAH [25], New York Online Access for Health, is useful if a person wants information in Spanish. Family Village [19], from the University of Wisconsin–Madison, is a wonderful Web site for people with disabilities. Besides teaching these sites, we link to them from the NAHEC links pages for both consumers and health professionals.

I also advise looking for online self-help groups. They're probably more useful to the consumer than a lot of the packaged information on the Web. It's through the mailing lists, discussion groups, and some of the personal sites that you really get into what it's like to live with a chronic disease.

It's like village life in the old days, when you would ask your aunt, your grandmother, your neighbor—but now your village is the globe.

If you are 1 of 20 people in the world with some rare syndrome, you can technically be in email communication with everyone else. In the past, the likelihood that anybody, particularly in a rural area, would run into someone else with a similar problem was nil. People need to share. And communities make a huge difference.

How would somebody find an online community?

The Self-Help Sourcebook Online [30] lists many of them, and Nursing & Health Care Resources on the Net has an extensive list of condition-specific mailing lists, in addition to the professional lists I mentioned earlier. You can also find online communities for disabilities in the "Library" section of Family Village. Once you're in the Library, click on the card catalog for "Specific Diagnoses." Once you've found the disorder, you can opt to find more information or to chat.

Do you have a feel for where this proliferation of health information is going? Ten years from now, what might we see?

I don't know if it will continue to grow or not. I think the newness is going to wear off for a lot of people, so the sites that are left are going to be of higher quality. I'd like to see more collaboration, like the HealthWeb project. I see a lot of peer-reviewed online journals without a subscription fee, and I wonder if we are going to see more of that.

There are future possibilities. Two nursing organizations have started fascinating projects, where nurse researchers register their research in progress with an abstract and so on. The Sigma Theta Tau International's Registry of Nursing Research [148] is a free service to members and subscription-based for others. The Canadian-International Nurse Researcher Database [125] is a free resource where nurses can register their research interests and contact information. This is the kind of thing that organizations should be looking toward promoting and developing.

Getting full-text information out to clinicians is also very important, and I hope that the day will come when the core medical journals and practice guidelines—all of them—are available electronically. As it is, fewer than 45 percent of the titles on my Key Nursing Journals chart are available electronically in full text from any source, and most of those for recent years only.

What about major frustrations?

My biggest frustration is looking at Web sites and trying to figure out where the organization is based, the date they put up the site—the basic authority behind the Web site.

I know what you mean. I'll look at a Web site and not be able to find a telephone number. These are sites that are professionally done; they're organizations that I know exist. They

spend a lot of money, and you have no way of contacting them except through email.

You also have no way of knowing how current the Web site is. We need to communicate more with Web editors. I put a notice out to several nursing lists saying that I was looking for particular standard information on Web sites; some of them actually fixed their sites as a result. Part of the shakedown that's going to occur is a whole new role for librarians in teaching critical thinking, as well as teaching people how to improve the credibility of their Web sites by including meta-tags and background information.

Critical thinking is key. It involves critical appraisal of the literature, being skeptical of what you read, and understanding that anybody can produce something on the Web. It involves understanding the importance of looking for authority and references, and the ability to evaluate what you're looking at and see what's behind it.

We need to teach students more about what peer review means and the editing cycle that articles undergo in order to be published in a peer-reviewed journal. If you do a general Web search on a disease, you get a much higher percentage of horror stories than if you look at the scientific literature as a whole. Somebody who has been hurt or damaged is much more likely to scream about it or say "poor me," than if she got through it okay with medical attention. The horror stories on the Web can be very scary. Even though these personal experiences are true, their numbers are out of proportion to the actual level of occurrence in the community. If you rely on reports from the Web, the risk looks worse.

But the anecdotal literature isn't going to go away.

Right, but it's out of proportion to reality. So, the next step is to become active partners with consumers, helping them take an active role in their own healthcare. This is a trend that the health field can't fight. Nursing has seen it for years. A lot of nursing theory revolves around working with patients, helping them do as much as they can for themselves. The medical model has been that the practitioner is God. Physicians who went to school with that as the model are having a heck of a time. Number one, it's difficult to be God when you can't always cure everything—you're setting yourself up for failure. Secondly, unless you're a super-specialist, you're never going to know as much about the patient's condition and response to that illness as the patient could learn in the long run. Doctors who want to work *with* the patients, to help them monitor their symptoms and communicate so they can get better care, are going to be way ahead in this trend.

Drawing on all your professional experience, what are the key things searchers should watch for?

Most importantly, if you are going to search a core of traditional online databases, it's crucial to know their unique features. The subject headings are different when you move from MEDLINE to CINAHL to PsycLIT. The subheadings are different. The age group headings are slightly different. You can use features in some databases that you can't in others. Use journal subsets to refine the information into something manageable and relevant to your patrons. Publication types in CINAHL and MEDLINE are different; using them correctly can provide really useful quality filters.

Knowing the full record is really important if you're going to be a super researcher; that is, knowing what you can get at through the indexing. You can't know all the features of every database, but if they do have special features, it's important to know them and use them. This is what you're paying for when you search a database versus the Web.

More broadly, we should be teaching health professionals how to request a search from a health science librarian, how to use library services when they're out in practice, and how to insist that they have access to such services. They should at least know, "Don't let your secretary or medical assistant call and make the search request. If it's important enough for us to do the search for you, it's important enough for you to call and spend two minutes talking about what you're looking for." The reference interview is absolutely crucial, but it takes two to do a good one.

Super Searcher Power Tips

➤ On searching allied health topics

I don't think there's any excuse for not using CINAHL. Some allied health fields, like music therapy and education, are better covered in PsycLIT. EMBASE picks up quite a lot in physical therapy. ERIC is strong in language and speech pathology, and any service provided by the school.

➤ On using tree structures in controlled vocabulary

You can go up and down the tree; if you're not getting enough with the term you've picked, you can go broader, or you can explode headings to get the narrower headings from underneath. Most good searchers prefer to be able to choose their own search method, depending on the question.

➤ On the value of online communities

Online self-help groups are probably more useful to the consumer than a lot of the packaged information on the Web. It's through the mailing lists and discussion groups and some of the personal sites that you really get into what it's like to live with a chronic disease. If you are 1 of 20 people in the world with some rare syndrome, you can technically be in email communication with everyone else. People need to share. And communities make a huge difference.

➤ On the problem of anecdoctal literature

If you do a general Web search on a disease, you get a much higher percentage of horror stories than if you look at the scientific literature as a whole. Somebody who has been hurt or damaged is much more likely to scream about it or say "poor me," than if she got through it okay with medical attention. Even though these personal experiences are true, their numbers are out of proportion. The risk is going to look worse.

➤ On making the most of traditional databases

It's key to know the unique features of the core group of databases you're searching. The subject headings are different when you move from MEDLINE to CINAHL to PsycLIT. The subheadings are different. The age group headings are slightly different. There are features you can use in some of the databases that aren't in others. You can't know all the features of every database, but if they do have special features, it's really important to know them and use them. This is what you're paying for when you go to a database versus searching the Web.

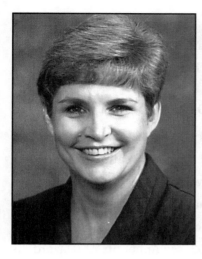

Auburn Steward

Assessing Toxic Risk

Auburn Steward, M.L.I.S., A.H.I.P., is the information specialist and reference librarian at the Center for Toxicology and Environmental Health on the University of Arkansas for Medical Sciences campus in Little Rock, Arkansas.

stewardauburn@exchange.uams.edu

Auburn, can you tell me a little bit about the Center?

We're a private incubator company for the University of Arkansas for Medical Sciences campus. We do environmental consulting and toxicology consulting, which includes things like risk assessment, industrial hygiene, and occupational health. Some of our people respond to chemical emergency situations.

How did you come to be the information specialist and reference librarian there?

I had been working for the Baptist Hospital library for about 15 years when the toxicologists I work for now contacted my former supervisor at the University of Arkansas Medical Sciences library. They asked her, based on what she knew about their business, whether she knew somebody who could set up a library, do their searching, and order their articles for them. She said, "Well, just about the only person I know who could cover all those bases would be Auburn." Meanwhile, I was looking for a change of scenery at that point, anyway, and had applied for the job. So they had heard my name before I even applied.

What kinds of searching do you do?

It varies from project to project. I do the toxicology side of medical, which might be related to an occupational incident or some environmental work that we're doing. For example, if we get an emergency response situation, I might be asked to get everything I can on a particular chemical. The first thing I do is jump online and get an HSDB [92, see Appendix A] (Hazardous Substances Databank) printout. That's not a bibliographic database, but a database of information about particular chemicals. You can search by chemical name, by the CAS (Chemical Abstracts Service) registry number, by its synonyms, and sometimes by product names. You get information about human health effects, emergency medical treatment, environmental fate, toxicity, and chemical safety, as well as answers to questions such as, "We've got this chemical on the ground; how do we clean it up?" Everything on a particular chemical is in one file; you can print the entire file or search and get just specific parts.

How do you access HSDB?

Through TOXNET [115], which is in the National Library of Medicine network. Some of the information comes from the Environmental Protection Agency (EPA) [87]. HSDB takes excerpts of information from other peer-reviewed sources; they'll say something like, "In *Goodman & Gilman* [182], here is what they say about this particular chemical," or "In this particular text, this is what was said about how toxic this chemical is." It takes information from all these other sources and compiles it into one database.

Is it also searchable by symptom? Can you ask, "This person must have come in contact with something; what could it have been?"

Yes, field searching is available, and there are several human toxicity fields. You could say, "Okay, let's search the human toxicity fields and see if nausea was one of the symptoms." Of course, you'll get a ton of chemicals with nausea as a symptom, but you could put in a cluster of symptoms to narrow it down.

I use the database that way, but for other kinds of questions. Let's say, for example, that some chemicals have been found on a piece of property. Of what chemical are those chemicals the degradation products? In other words, what chemical was there that degrades down into these other chemicals? Here, you search the biodegradation field for the chemicals you've found, and it tells you that these are biodegradation products of these other chemicals. Now you know what chemicals might have been used on that site. This is a real example of something that we have done in the past. A client is looking at a property for possible purchase; part of the process is a site assessment. They might do chemical soil sampling to see if it comes up with some kind of questionable chemical.

Do you ever get questions from companies that are considering using a substance in a product and want to know whether it's nontoxic?

Yes, a company was considering a particular chemical as the propellant in a medical formulation and wanted to know how that would work within their product. They were doing this in conjunction with a Food and Drug Administration approval. I provided the information to the toxicologist, who applied risk assessment methods to come up with the answer.

What other human health situations might come up?

Perhaps an individual has symptoms and says he was exposed to a certain chemical. Are these symptoms associated with an exposure to the chemical? If he's a painter and has memory loss after being exposed to such-and-such in the paint, has that chemical been documented to be toxic? We would use the MEDLINE [96] subheadings "adverse effects," "poisoning," or "toxicity." That is, here's the chemical, here are its adverse effects.

You can also start with a disease; you would use the subheadings "chemically induced" or "etiology." You ask, "Are there reports of this disease being chemically induced? Are there reports of this disease being induced by this chemical or these chemicals?" There are several ways to approach it, depending on exactly what the question is.

Reports exist that asbestos causes mesothelioma, an overgrowth of the lung lining. Reports exist that people have adverse reactions to latex gloves. People who do standard medical searching have run across these kinds of queries and probably don't even think of them as being toxicology questions. But toxicology can involve drug reactions, reactions to industrial or domestic products, or reactions to things in the environment. A very good article in *Occupational and Environmental Medicine* [63] entitled "Assessment of bibliographic databases performance in information retrieval for occupational and environmental toxicology" used the asbestos and latex examples to test various databases for toxicology coverage, to see how they compared and which gave the best retrieval.

What were the best databases?

The article was done by a group in France, which looked at BIOSIS [123], EMBASE [131], MEDLINE, NIOSHTIC [106], and TOXLINE [114]. For these particular topics, at least, over a two-year period, they concluded that TOXLINE is probably the most comprehensive. But they suggest that you ought to search a combination of TOXLINE and MEDLINE, or TOXLINE and EMBASE. They recommend a combination because no single database covers all the journals. We all know that some journals are not indexed completely in every database, so a journal indexed in MEDLINE might not have every article show up in TOXLINE; some of the articles on toxicity may not have made it into MEDLINE.

I also discovered that abstracts from conferences are not indexed in MEDLINE, but some of the databases that comprise TOXLINE do index conference proceedings, symposiums, and some textbooks. With a combination of databases, you get wider coverage of the toxicology literature.

What's the difference between TOXLINE and TOXNET?

TOXLINE is a bibliographic database made up of many different files from various sources. One section is TOXBIB, which takes toxicology information from MEDLINE. TOXLINE also includes references from BIOSIS and from NIOSHTIC, the National Institute of Occupational Safety and Health database. There's also information from the pharmaceutical literature, hazardous materials data, data from developmental and reproductive toxicology databases, and some citations to NTIS [107] documents. In recent years, they've added RISKLINE [120], a Swedish database of materials related to risk or toxicological effects.

TOXLINE is a combination of about 15 subfiles in all. You can search all of TOXLINE, or you can specify a particular part.

TOXLINE sounds like the equivalent of a vendor of toxicology literature.

Right. It was searchable through the National Library of Medicine directly or through Internet Grateful Med [91]. TOXLINE is now available on the Web through the TOXNET interface.

The databases accessible through TOXNET include the Hazardous Substances Databank, which I mentioned earlier; an

EPA database called IRIS (Integrated Risk Information System) [95]; RTECS (Registry of Toxic Effects of Chemical Substances) [113]; and GENE-TOX (Genetic Toxicology/Mutagenicity Data Bank) [90].

Some of these databases are also available through other sources. At one time, you could only search IRIS through TOXNET. IRIS is now at the EPA Web site, too. You can find NIOSHTIC and BIOSIS on Dialog [155].

With all the ways to get at these databases, where do you go for them?

My first choice is usually the TOXNET network. At one time the decision was to go directly to the MEDLARS program of the National Library of Medicine because it was cheaper than to search through Dialog. Now that it's on the Internet, it's free.

To what use do you put MEDLINE or EMBASE? Where do the medical literature databases fit in your work?

I use them to get an idea of whether there are any reports of a particular chemical being related to or causing a disease. Again, MEDLINE is good because you have those subheadings for "chemically induced" or "etiology" of the disease. EMBASE is similar to MEDLINE in many ways, but it does cover some of the foreign literature that MEDLINE doesn't. I'd start with MEDLINE because it allows you to be much more precise in your searching.

That's one of the drawbacks of TOXLINE. Because it's composed of so many different subfiles, there's no consistency among them. You can use the medical subject headings, or MeSH terms, but much of what you get when you do that is the same medical literature that you'll find in MEDLINE. So you have to supplement your medical headings with text-word searching and, if you've already searched MEDLINE, eliminate the TOXBIB section to avoid some of the duplication.

In other words, you'd start with MEDLINE, using controlled vocabulary and descriptors, then move to TOXLINE and eliminate the TOXBIB part?

That's one thing you can eliminate. On Internet Grateful Med, eliminating MEDLINE references is one of your choices. Also, when you're searching subject fields in TOXLINE on Internet Grateful Med, you're searching text-word fields of abstracts and complete documents in different subfiles, so your search is broader than it would be using medical headings. You have to adjust for that, weed through the results, and pick out the ones that look pertinent.

Which of the medical databases let you search by CAS numbers?

You can search by CAS number in MEDLINE, although not all the older records have CAS numbers. It's better to search in combination, with either a text word or a MeSH heading and the CAS number. BIOSIS and TOXLINE also have CAS numbers. Obviously the chemical databases have them.

When somebody comes to you and says, "I need a search," what do you ask them?

Since I work with basically the same people all the time, I've got them pretty well trained. They've gotten used to what I'm going to ask them. In some cases it helps for me to know the scope or the characteristics of the particular project, so I get a feel for what's needed.

I walk new researchers through a search request. After they've told me what they want, I repeat back to them my take on what they've said. I try to clarify how much information they want, whether they expect to find any information, or if they have an idea of how much there might be out there. Do they want to limit by years? Do they just want recent literature, maybe the last five or ten years, or do they want a comprehensive search? I try to focus them, to get them to think a bit harder about exactly what it is they are really asking for.

What if they tell you they expect to find something, and you don't find anything?

I go back to them and say, "Maybe I'm not using the right terminology, I'm not finding what I think are the correct things." I may take them some references and say, "This is what I'm finding; is this what you had in mind? If not, then explain it further, give me better terminology, give me synonyms. Maybe we need to broaden the search a bit and go back and try again." When I worked at the hospital, I told nursing students who would come in looking for information, "If you have to watch a surgery on this particular subject, you can be sure that there's some information out there about how the surgery is done. Just because you can't find it in the first place you look, don't give up, there are other sources." I tried to teach them that there's probably going to be information out there about almost anything they ask for.

In your kind of business, which is so crucial to human life, do you worry when you don't find anything? Maybe you missed something important. At what point can you consider a search finished?

That's a good question. I've been in that position a few times, but fortunately not in a life-crucial situation. I get requests like, "I want some information or studies on how this chemical affects the ecological system." Then, if I've tried TOXLINE and gone to Dialog and some of the environmental databases and I'm still not finding anything, I ask, "Well, here's the only thing that looks close, do you want me to keep looking?" I tell them what sources I've exhausted and leave the decision up to them.

Do you keep broadening the search so that you're not looking for problems specifically, but for anything to do with the substance?

I have done that, because you hate to fail. But I learned many years ago that sometimes they *want* no answer. Sometimes they want to know that nobody else has done something, so they can write it up. In the case of a spill, if that chemical's not listed in HSDB and we can't find anything in the Material Safety Data Sheets, maybe there isn't really a problem with that chemical. You have to look at it that way. Maybe there isn't any information because it's not a problem.

Do you use the Internet other than for access to TOXLINE or TOXNET?

Oh, all the time. My life depends on it these days. Doesn't everybody's? I get on one of the meta-search engines, and try to find what's out there that's not in the database literature. Sometimes you don't find much in the databases, and there's all kinds of information on the Internet. Some manufacturers include toxicity information on their Web sites. On a couple of sites, you can search MSDS-type sheets from a variety of companies. For example, at Cornell University [129], you can enter a chemical or a product name and get a variety of MSDS sheets from several manufacturers. How up-to-date they are is another question, but they do exist.

Do you ever use email or mailing lists for research?

I've done that a number of times, when I'm at my wit's end tracking something down. In one project, we needed to know the average intake of fluids in Germany. I found some information in a bibliographic database about a study that was done in Germany. I asked a question about this on MEDLIB-L [174], and a librarian in Germany eventually faxed me several pages of the study with information for various regions. MEDLIB-L covers a lot of the medical and related literature.

Do you get involved in sensitivity studies? For example, methyl methacrylate is used in bone cement and also in artificial nails. I had a client trying to figure out if someone who had a reaction to their artificial nails should or shouldn't have a total hip replacement done using bone cement.

That was an interesting one! We had a person who blamed his illness on exposure to something in his job. We were looking at what the causes of his symptoms might be. He had been allergy-tested, and it turned out that he was allergic to a lot of things other than what he might have run into in the workplace.

We have incidences in which people say, "Because such-and-such chemicals were released in the air by this plant down the road, I have all these diseases." They'll sit there with diabetes, heart disease, and all these things they've had for years, but suddenly it was caused by a particular chemical. The whole neighborhood is claiming that they were in some way injured by a chemical release which smelled bad. Part of our role might be to show that the odor threshold of a chemical—in other words, how soon you smell it—is much lower than the actual danger threshold of that particular chemical. Think about methane or sulphur; you can smell it long before you reach a level that's dangerous.

What changes do you see in the health/ toxicology area?

There is a lot more emphasis at the Environmental Protection Agency on the idea of risk-based risk assessments. When we do risk assessments, we are trying to determine what the current risk is for people who might be working or living on the site that's being cleaned up. Generally, risk assessment refers to an environmental risk to a group of people rather than to an individual. Once the site is cleaned up, what might be the adverse health effects on people living or working at that site? A higher level of cleanup is needed if people are going to live there than if the site is to be used as an industrial park or paved over for a parking lot.

How do you keep up professionally?

When I have a few minutes to spare, I visit certain job-related Web sites. I try to visit NIOSH, OSHA, EPA and others that might have new information that applies to what we're doing at work. I also visit a few library-related sites. Then I try to keep up with the newsletters and journals I still get in the mail. Those are useful for keeping my searching in line—alerting me to new fields that can be searched or that the structure of the database has changed in some way.

Earlier, you said that a lot of medical librarians are actually doing toxicity searching without realizing it. What would you suggest they do in order to do as comprehensive a job as possible, perhaps in the case of a poison control question?

Especially if their hospital does not have some kind of a poison index system, HSDB is good for that. HSDB includes an emergency treatment section taken from the Micromedex [167] Poison Index system. This provides not only emergency treatment information, but also very specific information about how it affects different systems of the body.

It also includes toxicity information: Here's the human toxicity of this particular chemical at different levels. We had one situation in which there was a spill of a chemotherapy agent, mytomycin-c, in a hospital. The first thing we did was look it up in HSDB and tell them, "This is what you need for cleanup, and this is the level of protective clothing you need to wear."

What other toxicity questions might a general medical researcher get into?

If they've looked up adverse effects of something, that's toxicology information. They might have a poisoning case. They may think they have an overdose of a drug and need to find the symptoms associated with that. So, they actually do toxicology searching without thinking about it in those terms.

How about some tips or tricks for using the resources you have to their fullest?

We have a lot of toxicology-related resources, including textbooks. I find it very useful to know the content of those resources. You can often find good information just by knowing what you have in-house. Start with that information and you won't necessarily have to jump online to find things. But once you do jump online, it's very important to know what kind of information is in what database and the structure of the databases. Knowing what's in HSDB, for example, helps you know that you can go there and find certain types of information. It's very important to be aware not just that the databases exist, but what kind of information they cover, their structure, and the best ways to search them.

Super Searcher Power Tips

➤ On what to search in a chemical emergency

The first thing is to jump online and get an HSDB (Hazardous Substances Data Bank) printout. That contains a lot of information about particular chemicals. You can search by CAS registry number, by name, by synonym, and sometimes by product name.

➤ On field searching in TOXNET

You could search the human toxicity fields and see if nausea was one of the symptoms. You could put in a cluster of symptoms to narrow it down. You could search the biodegradation field for the chemicals you've found, and it will tell you that these are biodegradation products of these other chemicals.

➤ On finding chemically-induced disorders

We would use the MEDLINE subheadings "adverse effects," "poisoning," or "toxicity." Here's the chemical, here are its adverse effects. Starting with a disease, you would use the "chemically induced" or "etiology" subheadings. Are there reports of this disease being induced by this chemical or these chemicals? There are several ways to approach it.

➤ On combining databases for toxicology searches

A group in France looked at BIOSIS, EMBASE, MEDLINE, NIOSHTIC, and TOXLINE. They concluded that if only one database is searched, TOXLINE is probably the most comprehensive. But they suggest using a combination of TOXLINE and MEDLINE, or TOXLINE and EMBASE, because not every database covers all the journals.

➤ On searching a poison control question

HSDB includes an emergency treatment section from the Poison Index portion of Micromedex. This not only gives emergency treatment information, but also very specific information about how it affects different systems of the body. It also has toxicity information: Here's the human toxicity of this particular chemical at different levels.

➤ On knowing your resources

You can often find good information just by knowing what you have in-house. Once you do jump online, it's very important to know not just that the databases exist, but what kind of information is in what database, the structure of the databases, and the best ways to search them.

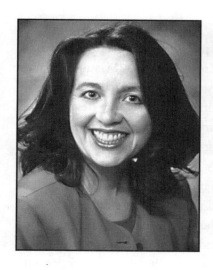

Nancy J. Allee

Finding Healthy Web Sites

Nancy J. Allee, M.P.H., M.L.S., is Director of Public Health Information Services and Access at the University of Michigan in Ann Arbor.

nallee@umich.edu

How did you get to your current job, Nancy, and what are your general duties?

My current job is my dream job, and I got here because I have both a library science degree and a public health degree. I worked in libraries in high school and college. Then I read *Megatrends* as a senior in college. That book talked about how important information specialists were going to be in the future, so I decided to get a degree in library science. My role models and my friends who went into librarianship were some of the brightest, most creative, and most socially responsible people I knew, so it seemed like a right choice.

My first job out of library school was a reference job at Northeastern State University in Oklahoma. Eventually, I had a chance to switch over to health sciences librarianship. The University is located in Tahlequah, which is a Cherokee word. My favorite definition of "Tahlequah" is "This will do." That's how I felt; it was my entry-level position, and would do as a good place to start my career. While I was in Tahlequah, the School of Optometry was doing a lot of research around the fact that

Native Americans as a group are predisposed to certain diseases, such as diabetes. I was very interested in health issues, so, after being the education and health sciences librarian, I worked on a Master's in public health. As soon as I finished my degree, a job opened at the public health library of the University of Michigan.

The current library is a merger of the information technology department and the library. It's a perfect combination of my areas of interest: information science and public health. Now I'm responsible for the network and computing area for the School of Public Health, as well as for classroom services, that is, audio-visual and room scheduling, and developing and maintaining the Web site. On the library side, we handle reference service, circulation, and collection management.

Who are your clients for reference services?

Our primary clientele is the School of Public Health and the faculty, staff, and students within the school, but we also work with other libraries on campus. We get lots of referrals, and we see undergraduates and graduate students from other programs with public health interests, such as the School of Social Work, the science library, and the Taubman Medical Library. We see clinicians, physicians, and research scientists from the medical school when they're researching an area that overlaps with public health.

What kinds of areas would those be? What would a public health library research that a biomedical library would not have?

A lot of the referrals that come from the medical school are for statistical information. They might be looking for some kind of health services research, perhaps statistics from various hospitals across the U.S. Recently, we've had people looking for policy and statutes information for emergency room physicians in instances of sexual assault; what are their reporting responsibilities? So, anything that speaks to statistical information or health management and policy information. People might be looking for epidemiology statistics, population statistics—comparative data of all sorts.

Where would you go for epidemiology information?

One project we're working on right now is to create a document or data center within the school. We're trying to build a set of databases relevant to the researchers here. Currently, we go to a government site that has census information, or to the National Center for Health Statistics [100, see Appendix A]. Those sites are great for national information, but often researchers and faculty are interested in Michigan data. So, we are trying to create a niche where we can provide electronic access to various kinds of Michigan data—for example, the Michigan hospital discharge data.

Michigan data is available to affiliated users of the school because our access to some of it is complicated by licensing agreements that are required to protect the confidentiality of the data. We collect vital statistics for each state for which this type of information is obtainable. Web sites such as the National Center for Health Statistics provide links to tabulated state data. Partners in Information Access for Public Health Professionals [110] provides a link to ASTHO [76] (Association of State and Territorial Health Officials) and the state data to which it provides access. There are workshops about creating Web interfaces to various data sets. EduCause [164], a professional organization that draws members from the library community as well as the information technology community, has a special interest group that looks at data.

You make a lot of data available on the Michigan Web sites. I've bookmarked the University of Michigan Document Center [172] because you can find almost any kind of publicly

available document through it. But you also have a metasite of medical megasites.

Yes. We call it the Megasite Project [12]. It's a metasite that compares health information megasites and search engines. We created it for health information professionals and other interested users who are trying to find the best resources on the Web for various kinds of health information.

My colleague, Pat Anderson, and I began working on the project as part of a special task force. We're about three years into the project. It started as an outgrowth of a project from HealthWeb [4], which began as a collaborative effort by a group of librarians in the Midwest region of the U.S. who were trying to get a handle on the World Wide Web and how much information was out there. They wanted to provide access to evaluated, noncommercial, health-related information resources on the Internet. From the beginning, one of HealthWeb's defining features has been its decision not to be comprehensive, but to evaluate and select reliable, quality sites that people could be confident in using.

One of the projects that emerged was finding out who else was trying to evaluate information on the Internet. Our task force was formed to find other sites similar to HealthWeb. We tried to approach it in a systematic way but, as everyone knows, information changes daily on the Web as new sites are created and others disappear. Our colleagues on HealthWeb started sending us pointers to sites as they became aware of them. We built our list of sites and then went about defining and trying to develop an assessment tool to evaluate them.

So you're evaluating Web sites that purport to evaluate Web sites.

Yes. We did the first phase of the project and reported at several conferences. The feedback was very positive. Once the Megasite was created, librarians told us that they used it as a resource for their library school classes in medical librarianship. The general public wrote and told us that they thought this was a very valuable thing to do. We went back to the HealthWeb board with this feedback, and HealthWeb has decided to incorporate the Megasite Project into the HealthWeb pages.

Were you able to draw any conclusions about that great morass of information you found?

We learned that there are many very, very good sites in the area of health and medical information. We discovered that it is challenging to stay on top of all the new sites that are being created. It is a huge and complex task to identify sites and develop criteria to evaluate them. Our evaluation instrument is something that we're constantly working on to improve.

We also learned that, in general, if you want very current information or information on a topic that's been getting attention recently, you can use a general search engine and be just as successful as if you're using a health information search engine.

That's almost contrary to popular belief!

Yes. It was surprising to us, but it's also a compliment to those general search engines and what they are able to do.

Does that hold true specifically for topics that are in the public eye at the moment?

Yes, as well as for consumer health information. If it's recently released and you heard about it on some TV news program or the radio, the general search engines do a great job of linking to those results. Another thing we discovered is that, if it's a well-defined topic and has been of interest for a while, almost any search engine should produce good results.

What about the more obscure or technical topics?

For those—especially if you're looking for information that has passed through a rigorous peer-review process and adheres to scientific standards—you'll want to look for official health information sites. Also, if you want to avoid so-called "adult" content, which is a concern for some people, using a health information site prevents you from pulling up a lot of links to inappropriate material. That's an added value to using sites that focus specifically on health information. You don't always anticipate some of the connotations of the terminology you're using. We ran into a problem when we tested various search engines using the word "stroke." For us, the word had only a medical aspect, but some of the results we got were very, very surprising.

We found that the only sites that gave clinically appropriate answers to the toughest clinical questions were health information sites. So, for clinicians, the health information sites might be a first point of reference. It's very important to define your topic carefully, think through your question, and know who your target audience is. Depending on whether you need information for a patient or a clinician, then you might choose a specific site in accordance with the target.

What would you look for in a consumer site?

We look at whether the site identifies its target audience—that it clearly states whether it's designed for clinicians, students, practitioners, librarians, or the general public. We look at whether the site provides information about how they select the resources that they link to, and who is doing the selection. We look at the update frequency, so we can be confident in knowing that someone is administering the site and providing quality control for it. We also look at whether navigational assistance is provided and the ease of navigability—whether a person who's searching the site has to scroll through numerous pages to find where they can type in their search question.

How would you evaluate a site for a clinician?

We found that many of the clinically-oriented sites require registration. That is one way to signify that they are indeed targeted to health professionals. They try to track their search activity to provide better service, and they enable users of that site to customize the way they search it. So, one thing to note for a clinician would be whether the site requires registration, because that can carry a lot of meaning.

Another area where you could make a distinction is between a consumer's patience and a physician's. In the focus groups I've done with physicians at the medical school, they emphasize again and again the limited amount of time they have for searching the Web. They want an interface that is very user-friendly and straightforward. Those kinds of navigational issues would be important to both audiences, but may be more important to a clinician audience.

What do you think the Web is particularly good for overall?

For reference librarians at PHISA and myself, it is the statistical and government information that's available. The role that the government has taken in migrating so much of its information to the Web has meant a tremendous improvement for us in the service we can provide to users. We can link them to those resources, and they can be assured in knowing that they're getting reliable information, that they can have confidence in the statistics they're looking at. Our research is showing us that the Web is getting better and better all the time as a resource for consumers, and that there is a lot of good information out there, if you define a search strategy that gets you there efficiently.

Your project is geared toward evaluating sites for other people. What do you look for personally?

We look for quick response, servers that aren't slow, that the session doesn't expire and lose your search results before you're finished looking through them. Often, we'll want to bookmark a particularly useful search result, especially if it's information that we had difficulty finding and we anticipate that the question may come up again on the reference desk. So we want the search results to have titles that are meaningful. When we look through our bookmarks we need to see terminology, keywords, or something that clues us in to what those results are. If we're pulling together a pathfinder on a particular topic area and citing information that may be helpful, we'll include the URLs of the results of specific searches.

Can you describe a pathfinder?

A pathfinder is a quick reference guide to information on a particular subject. I have one in front of me from the Patient Education Resource Center at the Cancer Center here at the University of Michigan. I'll just go through it to give you an idea of what a pathfinder might include.

It has a very short, bulleted definition of the Internet. This was designed as a consumer information resource, so the target audience here would be patients using the Cancer Center library. It has a section on the World Wide Web, and under that, links to recommended Web sites. It gives the URLs for the American Cancer Society's Web page [70], CancerNet [84], Oncolink [26], the Cancer Center library itself, and the University of Michigan Cancer Center [171] for more information. There's a section for email and chat, which mentions several email lists and chat rooms. Then it gives tips for evaluating Internet sites—who's providing the information, whether it's a university, a government agency, or a commercial company. It advises people to read the "About Us" section so they can determine whether it's a reputable site, and to look at whether charges are assessed for searching this site. Finally, it has an advisory section that quotes *Consumer Reports* about how frequently information on the Internet changes—it's important for this reason that the pathfinder itself carries the date when it was last updated—and an advisory statement about making sure you consult with your doctor about any information you have a question about.

Okay, if somebody handed you a topic and said, "I need you to create a pathfinder on this," where do you start?

We look at a combination of traditional resources and Internet resources. We go through our reference collection, then use the online catalog and run some searches on the topic, limiting it to our collection. We then evaluate the ones that seem to offer the most information on the topic. Then we look at the few stand-alone CD-ROM workstations that we still have, and include information about those that would be relevant. Then we go to the Internet. We start with resources that are familiar to us, so we go to HealthWeb and see if ours is one of the subject areas included on that site. We go to our Megasite Project and see if there are sites that provide information in that area.

Then we link from the Megasite Project to search engines we found to be the best for Boolean searching. Depending on the topic, we will probably run the search in those search engines and then go through the process of evaluating those results.

Nancy, you also do reference work. When you've completed your research, how do you deliver the results to your patrons?

A lot of people now interact with us electronically through our reference desk's email address. We send results in the form of URLs, usually with an annotation explaining how a site is going to be able to help them answer the question, what they can expect to find there, the years and scope of coverage, and who is providing the information. We also fax information. A unit within the university library system called MITS, the Michigan Information Transfer Service, provides document delivery to users all over the world. It's a fee-based service, but if someone needs something, they will mail or fax it to them. For people who prefer print, if it's not a lot of pages, we'll print it out and leave it in our patron pick-up box. But a lot of our interaction is through email.

What about the full text of journal articles?

We point people to the full text. For example, we have access to the Ovid [158] version of MEDLINE [96], and our licensing agreement with Ovid gives us access to full-text resources. So we point people to Medsearch in Ovid, give them our search strategy so they can reproduce it if they want to, and give them the journal citation. They can go into the full-text resources to print it out.

An issue that arises there—as I'm sure it does for other institutions that have distance-education students—is what form of authentication is used for access to these electronic resources. At Michigan, we have been using IP authentication, which is a barrier for distance learners. It particularly affects us in PHISA, because the School of Public Health does have a distance education program, the On Job/On Campus program. It's for professionals who want to work on a Master's in public health and have a limited amount of time because they're working full time. Our challenge has been to come up with ways to provide them with access to these resources, because we don't want to differentiate between what they and the residential students have access to. It involves investing in a proxy server, which allows you to use other methods of authentication. In the near future, we will have a system where people can authenticate by their unique name.

If you could blue-sky, what resources would you like to see available that aren't?

That's a good question. In the area of public health specifically, I'd like easier access to the gray literature—reports, policy statements, newsletter articles, professional association materials, and especially all kinds of agency reports. It would be a dream world to have easy access to those.

I'd also like to have comparative data, nationally and internationally. To give you a specific example, when I came here I spent a good year trying to get a resource called *African Index Medicus*, because of the information that it was indexing in the area of HIV and AIDS in African countries. We were completely unsuccessful in our efforts to purchase that resource through standard means of acquisition. What eventually happened is that WHO, the World Health Organization, provided access from their Web pages. That made a tremendous difference in the kind of reference service we could provide for people who were looking for international data.

I'd like more statistical and epidemiological data, not only at the state level but at the county level. That would be a tremendous, tremendous resource for our researchers here. I see steps in that direction, but I think it will be a very complex process. If states and counties could provide that information via the Web, could promote it and make people aware that it exists, it would be a huge step in the right direction.

Is the role of the librarian changing?

The skills that are needed are changing in some ways, but not the role. The more sophisticated a user of technology you are, the better service you can provide, and the better contribution you can make to the profession. Four years ago, the first step in doing a reference search would be to look at the print collection. Now, the first step is going to the Internet. The tools are changing; the necessary skill set is changing.

In terms of the role, we're finding that the librarian is as essential as he or she has ever been. There is a lot of information out there. Librarians have the skills to know the appropriate subject headings—and, if they don't know, they experiment until they can determine them. They can understand and evaluate content. That—and being able to define a search strategy that allows people to get to that content—is critical. It's as critical as ever.

Super Searcher Power Tips

➤ On finding statistical data

Web sites such as the National Center for Health Statistics provide links to tabulated state data. The Partners in Information Access for Public Health Professionals site provides a link to ASTHO (Association of State and Territorial Health Officials) and the state data to which it provides access. EduCause, a professional organization that draws members from the library community as well as the information technology community, has a special interest group that looks at data.

➤ On the value of general search engines

In general, if it's recently released and you heard about it on some TV news program or the radio, the general search engines do a great job of linking to those results. If it's a well-defined topic and has been of interest for a while, almost any search engine should produce good results.

➤ On the value of a health-specific search engine

For information that has passed through a rigorous peer-review process and adheres to scientific standards, you want to look for official health information sites. Using a health information site prevents you from pulling up a lot of links to inappropriate content. We found that the only sites that gave clinically appropriate answers to the toughest clinical questions were health information sites. So, for clinicians, the health information sites might be a first point of reference.

➤ On what makes a good site

We look at whether the site identifies its target audience—that it clearly states whether it's designed for clinicians, students, practitioners, librarians, or the general public. We look at whether it provides information about how they select the resources that they link to, and who is doing the selection. We look at the update frequency, so we can be confident in knowing that someone is administering the site and providing quality control for it. We also look at whether navigational assistance is provided and the ease of navigability.

➤ On creating a topic-specific pathfinder

We look at traditional resources as well as Internet resources. We go through our reference collection, then use the online catalog, limiting it to our collection. Then we go to HealthWeb, and to our Megasite Project. Then we link to search engines we found to be the best for Boolean searching. Depending on the topic, we will run the search in those search engines, and then go through the process of evaluating those results.

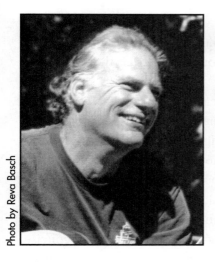

Alan Eshleman

Online Patient Liaison

Alan Eshleman, M.D., is a practicing physician with Kaiser Permanente and National Physician Lead for KP Online.

doctore@well.com

Alan, you play several different roles for Kaiser Permanente. Can you tell me about that?

I've been with Kaiser for about 12 years. Until fairly recently, I was a traditional internist with an office practice and a large group of patients. I taught house staff and occasionally attended on the hospital wards. In October 1999, I began diversifying, reduced the amount of clinical time I spent, and went to work for KP Online. That's Kaiser's new members-only Web site project. Now, I spend half my time working on KP Online and the other half seeing patients. That was one of the conditions of the KP Online job; they wanted somebody who was still doing clinical medicine. That was a really good idea on their part, because if you stray too far from the actual hands-on practice of clinical medicine, into writing or media medicine, you can sometimes lose sight of what it's really like.

Now I'm the National Physician Lead, which amounts to being the medical director for the Web site project. I recruit and train other people in the organization to moderate online discussion groups and help pilot ideas for Web-based projects that involve interaction between healthcare providers and patients. I also do quality-assurance work on the materials that we put out on our Web site.

KP Online is an official outreach of our medical group, and although we are very adamant that we're not dispensing medical care and treatment, we *are* giving advice, counsel, and explanations about medical problems, how to seek medical care, and the like. So, we periodically review what we put out on the Web site. We want to make sure that the advice or information conforms to the highest contemporary standards of medical practice; that the actual quality of the postings and writing is clear, concise, and responsive to the members' questions; and that it stimulates further discussion. I also monitor six or seven of the discussion groups and actually contribute to and write for them.

Are these actual discussion groups or are they queries from KP's client base?

They're actual discussion groups, although they tend to gravitate toward being Q&A sessions. Right now, there are about 30 topics on our board covering such things as women's health, men's health, chronic disease, pediatrics, and organizational issues, like "How do I get this from Kaiser?" or "How can I contact my physician more efficiently?" Some of the topics really take off on their own. For instance, there's a fairly active breast cancer topic that has largely turned into a self-sustaining support group.

But you still have to monitor the groups.

Right. These boards need almost no input from the professionals unless they ask, or unless there's something that we really think needs to be commented on. But we have to monitor them to make sure that no bogus information is going out and also just to make sure that no flame wars develop.

Typically, I'm writing for a discussion group like Chronic Disease or General Health that tends to be more Q&A. People are told something by their doctor and, when they get home, realize that they aren't quite sure what they were told. They come online and ask, "My doctor said I had Reynaud's Syndrome; what is that really?" If I think it has broad enough appeal, I'll answer it and, occasionally, I will encourage people to go off the board and email me directly. Some things are better handled in email.

What is the role of email in physician-patient interaction?

On the discussion board, if they're talking about personalities and naming names, it can be problematic. When somebody initiates their complaint in that kind of format, it's impossible to respond to them online. Medical ethics standards prevent the physician who's been accused from discussing specifics of the case in a discussion group. So, I strongly encourage members with an important complaint to just send it to me, and I will make sure that it gets to somebody. That's pretty much a stopgap solution; in time, I think we must have some sort of direct email communication between members and their physicians.

But I definitely see physician-patient email as a direction in providing information. Right now, the major resistance is coming from the providers who are worried that they're going to be inundated with messages. That's not an unrealistic worry, considering what the telephone does to them now, but the demand for email is very strong. It is the number-one demand from the members. They want to know how they can communicate directly with their doctor by email. We're trying to come up with a system, but we can't do it yet. A lot of physicians are, in fact, communicating with their patients by email, but only on a case-by-case basis.

You said that one of your tasks is training. How do you train the KP Online members to find information?

We have one discussion group on the Kaiser board called "Finding Answers on the Internet." There, I've been concentrating on three different places to send people. I use PubMed [112, see Appendix A] a lot, Healthfinder [3], and then any of their favorite search engines like Yahoo! [153], Infoseek [151], Lycos [152], or whatever. Working with a small set of those resources, I get fairly interactive with the patients. For example, one California patient was a pregnant diabetic, which is a special risk group. She said, "I can't find any information about Sweet Success." Sweet Success is a nationwide program for improving pregnancy outcomes for diabetic women. I went to Infoseek, did a search on "Sweet Success diabetes California," and, of course, it returned several hits. I went back to the conference and said, "Here's the information that you seek, and here's how I did it." I just basically laid it out—step one, step two, step three, step four, here's what happened, thank you very much. There's a member who's probably not going to ask a question like that again, because now she knows how to do it herself.

Sometimes, the question will be a little bit more complicated, like "How do I find out about all the cancer research protocols being run in the United States?" Then I may direct them to the NIH [102] Web page, since they administer this sort of thing. I'll tell them to use the NIH search engine for clinical trials, ClinicalTrials.gov [85].

Is consumer searching changing your practice?

A lot of the members who come to KP Online have already figured out how to search. They're coming and saying, "I found this on the Internet; what do you think of it?"

It's changing parts of our practice. I don't think that the Internet revolution, or whatever you want to call it, is really going to transform medicine. The day-in and day-out medicine in the trenches hasn't changed all that much, but you do see more people coming in with a sheaf of printouts from the Web and asking what you think of it, or coming to you with perhaps more knowledge of a subject than you would have expected your average patient to have. So, to that extent, it has changed the practice. If somebody comes to me and hands me a bunch of information about a health condition and asks, "What do you think?", at the very least I'm going to have to look it over and tell them what I think.

Sometimes, though, the sites they're going to also carry lots of advertising. That's fine, but the direct-to-consumer drug ads are a big headache for all of us in practice. They generate false expectations; for example, patients demanding Relenza for "flu" when they don't have anything other than a common cold.

But overall, the Internet is creating a more knowledgeable patient.

What about all the false information that's out there?

There's a lot of false information circulating. But there's been a lot of false information circulated through other means, like your friendly neighborhood health food store pushing the supplement of the week. That's been going on since long before the Internet. In fact, those people have just moved their practices onto the Internet, where they're getting wider distribution. But, yes, patients do come to me with fairly hokey things that they've downloaded from the Internet. Usually it's from a commercial site, and usually it's asking for money. I tell them to beware of sites that ask for your money.

Where would you tell people to go if they're not Kaiser members? For example, what do you look for in a consumer information site?

I look for the standard admonition that none of this is a substitute for real face-to-face medical care by a human being, and I look for ease of navigation. The admonition I look for is a simple statement that "None of the information displayed on this site is meant to be a substitute for diagnosis or treatment by a licensed physician or other practitioner. If you are experiencing symptoms or have other concerns about your personal health, please see a physician as soon as possible."

I also like a really good search engine that will take keywords that are not too jargony, so a person without a whole lot of experience in searching or a lot of background in medicine can actually get to where he or she is going.

"Heart attack" instead of "myocardial infarction"?

Right, heart attack. And call a stroke a stroke instead of a cerebrovascular accident, and call a cold a cold instead of an upper respiratory infection. You can cross-index things like that, but make it real simple. That's part of what I meant by "ease of navigation"—a minimum of jargon. If a reasonably intelligent layperson goes to a site and cannot find information about a common health problem—either because the information isn't there or because it's classified according to an unfamiliar term—something's wrong.

It's also important to show updating. I always worry when I go to a site that hasn't been changed since 1997. Medical information should be updated fairly frequently. The editor in me cringes when I see postings that are sloppily edited, with a lot of spelling mistakes. I like sites where some thought has been given to what the page looks like to the eye. I think DrKoop.com [18] is very good about that. I send a lot of people to that site. It's a fairly nicely designed Web page, it has a great deal of stuff from a consumer point of view, and it has a lot of chat.

At one point, Dr. Koop's site took some well-deserved criticism for presenting what was advertising as a news story, but it remains a useful site for laypeople. There are a whole bunch of sites—like InteliHealth [22], CBSHealthwatch [17], Onhealth [27], and the public areas of WebMD [32]—that all blur together, with hot-off-the-presses medical news, "ask the doctor" features, scheduled chat events, and support areas.

None of these sites pays much attention to the fact that getting medical care is expensive and difficult for millions of people. Also, their advice seems geared to an imaginary "patient," who is still getting care within a traditional, private-practice model.

You mentioned earlier that consumers should beware of sites that ask for money.

Right. I disapprove of the ones that take advantage of a patient who comes from the doctor's office, devastated by the news that he's got prostate cancer. He goes home, turns on the computer, and does a search on prostate cancer. He finds Rejuva.com or something. Here's a site with a couple of pages of text that talks about prostate cancer in very nonscientific or pseudo-scientific terms. Then you scroll down to find that it's saying that this herbal-whatever is available for three easy payments of $39.95 a month. They don't exactly say it will cure prostate cancer, because that's illegal; but they say everything short of that. They are basically selling a worthless product.

There are sites all over the Web now that purport to sell all manner of powerful hormones as a cure for aging. It doesn't work, it takes a lot of people's money, and sometimes it delays getting them the kind of care that might actually help them.

I'm not the world's biggest proponent of mainline Western medicine; I think that it has its failings, too. I just have seen enough examples of people faced with a serious diagnosis who have leapfrogged over a serious discussion with their physicians and gone directly to the Web or a health food store and paid good money for an essentially worthless product.

Of course, if you went to PubMed, that wouldn't be a problem. If you go to Infoseek, it *is* a problem. If you ask PubMed about prostate cancer, you'll be overwhelmed with scientific journals. If you go to Infoseek, most of the returns are going to be commercial sites.

Something I look for in a site is whether it tells me where the information is coming from.

That's a very good point. I caution people to beware of sites that don't reference their statements. There are some pretty outlandish and unreferenced statements that read like chain letters. They don't give the date or tell who it is, but they'll say something like "Dr. Smith of New York has used this oil to remarkable effect." Oh, really? Who's Dr. Smith? Where is he in New York?

How would you find out who this doctor really is?

If you can't run the statement to ground, be very, very worried about it. Most state medical boards now have public access Web sites that list the names and licensure status of physicians in that state. Some states even release information about which practitioners have been subject to discipline, revocation of their licenses, and even criminal charges. Most reference libraries have copies of *The Directory of Medical Specialists* [37], which lists all the board-certified practitioners in the country. Also, almost every county has a local medical society. You can call and ask for help in checking credentials. For example, the Medical Board of California [118] has a site where you can verify a physician's licensure.

Considering how much misinformation is out there, how do you decide what terms to use in a general search engine?

Instead of asking about a disease in particular, or adding modifiers like "cure" or "treatment," the best thing to do is ask for organizations. If you want to know about diabetes, search for diabetes organizations. If you want to know about prostate cancer, or breast cancer, or lupus, or rheumatoid arthritis, search for organizations. By and large, most of the foundations or organizations that are devoted to specific diseases supply links to fairly reliable literature and to fairly reputable practitioners, medical organizations, and medical centers. Healthfinder's very good at finding those organizations.

When you can't answer a question out of your own experience, what do you do?

I've got about 40 people who have agreed to act as consultants. If I can't answer a member question out of my own experience, I'll try to determine what specialty would be best equipped to deal with it, and I'll email the inquiry to one of my consultants.

You search your human database.

Yes. Our concept is, we are building the virtual medical center. People enjoy knowing that the response they're getting is from somebody they could actually see if they really wanted to. That's my brain trust, the virtual medical center.

If there's something I really can't find any information about, and the consultants don't know, and I'm just coming up with zeros, I must admit that I call my friend who's the medical librarian at the medical center. If it's to be found, she'll find it. That's her job.

Super Searcher Power Tips

➤ On the need for accuracy in disseminating information

We periodically review what we put out on the Web site. We want to make sure that the advice or information conforms to the highest contemporary standards of medical practice, that the actual quality of the postings and writing is clear, concise, and responsive to the members' questions, and that it stimulates further discussion.

➤ On electronic physician-patient interaction

I definitely see physician-patient email as a direction in providing information. It is the number-one demand from members. They want to know how they can communicate directly with their doctor by email. A lot of physicians are, in fact, communicating with their patients by email, but only on a case-by-case basis.

➤ On what to look for in a consumer site

I look for the standard admonition that none of this is a substitute for real face-to-face medical care by a human being, and I look for ease of navigation. The admonition I look for is a simple statement that "None of the information displayed on this site is meant to be a substitute for diagnosis or treatment by a licensed physician or other practitioner. If you are experiencing symptoms or have other concerns about your personal health, please see a physician as soon as possible."

➤ On the need for simple language

I like a really good search engine that will take keywords that are not too jargony, so a person without a whole lot of experience in searching or a lot of background in medicine can actually get to where he or she is going. If a reasonably intelligent layperson goes to a site and cannot find information about a common health problem—either because the information isn't there or because it's classified according to an unfamiliar term—something's wrong.

➤ On determining a physician's credentials

Most state medical boards now have public access Web sites that list the names and licensure status of physicians in that state. Some states even release information about which practitioners have been subject to discipline, revocation of their licenses, and even criminal charges. Most reference libraries have copies of *The Directory of Medical Specialists*, which lists all the board certified practitioners in the country. Also, almost every county has a local medical society. You can call and ask for help in checking credentials.

➤ On using a general search engine to research diseases

Instead of asking about a disease in particular, or adding modifiers like "cure" or "treatment," the best thing to do is ask for organizations. If you want to know about diabetes, search for diabetes organizations. Most of these foundations or organizations that are devoted to specific diseases supply links to fairly reliable literature and to fairly reputable practitioners, medical organizations, and medical centers.

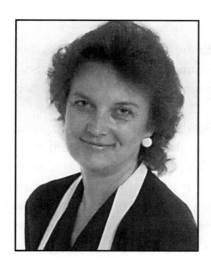

Pam Geyer

Focused on the Consumer

Pam Geyer, M.B.A., is President of MEDcetera, Inc., a medical information service that provides customized research reports on specific medical topics.

pgeyer@netropolis.net

Pam, you've been conducting healthcare research for consumers for several years. What's your background, and how did MEDcetera come about?

I worked as a medical technologist for a number of years in hospital laboratories. Then, I went back to school and got an M.B.A. in health services administration. Following that, I worked as a market researcher for what is now Frost & Sullivan. While I was there, an Israeli friend of mine wanted to do consumer medical information in Israel, and she asked me to help her do some market research on what it would take to set it up. While she was visiting me in the United States, we went out together and interviewed people. Ultimately, she decided against the idea, instead setting up a medical library at Hadassah Hospital in Israel. But I set up this service in California. I took it on part time, and sort of eased out of market research and into consumer medical research. I've been doing it for about nine years.

In 1991, it seemed to be a time of opportunity, just before people became aware of medical information that they could get online. People were not yet using the Internet to the extent they are now. There weren't many commercial sites back then. So, I saw an opportunity to educate people about getting information about their medical conditions.

I was very fortunate to get a lot of early publicity. I was interviewed by the medical doctor on the local NBC station for a three-minute medical segment. When it aired, they got so many calls at the station that they ran it three more times with my phone number. Then they sent the program on to the network, and it was on NBC Nightside News, a late night news show, as well as the local affiliate stations. So, I got a lot of publicity in the first six months of my business.

Who are your clients now?

I've stayed with serving the consumer. Whether that's smart or not remains to be seen, but that's where my passion lies. I have done some work for companies, but I really like helping people. I don't make nearly as much money as somebody who works for businesses, though. The consumer can't afford to pay as much. But I really enjoy helping people this way. I have supplemented the consumer work with doing market research or other kinds of searching for corporations.

When consumers come to you, how much of your service do they understand?

That's a good question. It depends on how they find me. If they've found me through an article that mentions my business, they have some idea, but they want to know how it works. Likewise, if a friend has told them, they usually have some idea. I get a lot of clients by word of mouth. But if somebody calls cold and asks, "How does your service work?", I'll explain a standard search, which is a MEDLINE [96, see Appendix A] search. I tell them that I can do other kinds of searching, but this is the basic level. Some people will want a more extensive search, perhaps with alternative medicine aspects. The price varies, depending on what they want and how long I think it will take. I always give them a quote ahead of time.

"Repeat clients," or people who have been referred by somebody who has used the service, usually say, "I need to find out what treatments there are for aneurysm" or "arterial blockage" or whatever condition they have. They sometimes ask me how much it costs, but often they know, and they know what they're going to get.

Somebody called me recently and asked, "What do you do?" After I told him, he said, "Well, this is for a friend of mine. How much do you charge?" I told him, and he said, "Well, this is what he's got. He can't urinate." When I asked for the diagnosis, he said, "The doctor just told him he couldn't urinate." I said, "Well, I really need to have a diagnosis." His response was, "Well, that's what I'm calling you about." I said, "We don't give a diagnosis. We just give medical information. We can do a search on treatments if you have a diagnosis, but I still need to have a diagnosis." In the end, he said he would tell his friend about this.

Now, I don't know whether this really was for a friend or whether I'll ever hear from him again, but that's the kind of thing you pick up on. My intuition told me that this guy didn't quite understand, didn't really want to understand, and maybe didn't want to pay for it. I don't know. But he was not somebody I would encourage to go through with using the service.

Can they generally tell you what it is that they want to know the treatment for?

Occasionally, somebody will not have a diagnosis, and I usually ask them to call their doctor and get one. I really need a diagnosis. I need to know what the doctor said they have, so that I know I'm getting them the right information. Many symptoms overlap a lot of different diseases.

How does your reference interview go?

I try to get as much information about them and their condition as I can. I ask who the search is for—is it for themselves or for somebody else, and if so, is it male or female? I ask their age. I try to get the exact diagnosis, how it relates to their age and their sex, if there are any complicating factors, anything their doctor has told them about it that might be relevant. If it's cancer, I ask them what stage it's in and what cell type it is. These are all qualifying questions when I go to do the search. Sometimes, a person will be really vague and I won't know exactly why; I think they want it for themselves, but they'll pretend it's for somebody else. Sometimes, if they haven't been really forthcoming, I have to call them back and say, "Look, I need some more information."

I guide the interview based on what they're saying. If they say, "I want to find the treatment for acne," I might ask them, "Is this for you or is it for a son or daughter?" If it's for a son or daughter, I ask, "How old?", because sometimes that makes a difference. Then I ask what treatments they have tried, and what treatments their doctor has recommended. I don't always use all the information I ask for, but I like to know as much as I can, so that if I get 500 citations, I can narrow it down a little bit better.

For something like this, where the client needs to know what treatments exist for a particular disease, where do you look?

I use MEDLINE if they want a standard search. You have to remember that consumers do not have a lot of money, and they want everything they can find. So, I always tell them that this is the best; this is peer-reviewed. I often get the question, "Will I be able to understand what it says?" I tell them two things—First, that it's an overview of what's been published on the treatment of their condition in the last couple of years, and they should look through the titles and mark the ones that sound relevant. Then, if they can't understand the abstract—I call it the "summary"— the last two or three sentences will usually summarize the research in lay terms. Secondly, I suggest that, after they've looked it over and marked it up, they should take it to their doctor and get the doctor's opinion.

I really coach the consumer client to have a dialogue with the doctor rather than a confrontation. I suggest that they say something like, "You know, when you told me I had this condition, I wanted to find everything out about it that I could, and I found this research service and they sent me this, and I really want you to look at it and give me your opinion on it." Doctors can easily be intimidated if you go in and say, "Well, what do you think about this? Why didn't you tell me about this?"

But I think of a doctor as a consultant. If you ask consultants to help with your business, you pay them a lot of money and they tell you what to do. Then, you use your judgment about whether or not it will work for your business. Most of the time, if they're good consultants, you do what they say. I like to look at doctors that way. We are hiring them to give us their expertise on how to keep our health or get our health back. It's a different perspective than going to doctors and putting our health in their hands and doing whatever they tell us to do. It's a paradigm shift. So, I try to coach people if they're open to that approach.

What about people who want to do the research themselves?

There has been a shift in the last few years toward people who are fascinated with the Internet, wanting to do their own research. At the same time, so much on the Internet is commercial in nature. Unless you have a discerning eye, you can't always tell. In fact, a lot of my more recent clients are people who are computer-savvy and know that they can't get it on their own, or that they want an expert to do it. So, when people call me and ask, "Can't I find this myself?", I tell them, "Of course you can, especially now that PubMed [112] is available. But if you really want a good quality search, you might want to think about having somebody else do it." I don't try to sell the service to people who call and say, "Well, why can't I find this on the Internet myself?" I just tell them what I think and let them decide.

Once you've done a standard search, what would the next step be? Where do you go when a patient says, "This is all very well and good, but I want the next level of research."

I don't often get people coming back and asking for the next level, which I think says something about MEDLINE. But there are times when I will suggest it myself. Then I look at reputable medical sites on the Internet. After a search, people often call me back and ask for a few articles, and I will usually use a document delivery service to get them.

What about the various cancer sites, such as PDQ [111]?

I use PDQ, as well as some sites for clinical trials of cancer. It depends on how much information people want. What I like about PDQ is it gives you an overview of the cancer in all its stages, and what the standard treatments are. It's fast reading. When I do a cancer search, I do two parts, the PDQ and then the MEDLINE search.

Do you use the MeSH terms and headings for searching?

I generally search by MeSH terms. I really like the command language version of MEDLINE. I think PubMed is very cumbersome; if you have a complex search, it's hard to use. When I was using ELHILL—the command language version direct to the National Library of Medicine—I would have searches that might be 10 to 20 search statements long. PubMed just isn't geared to that. It's built for quick-and-dirty searches. You lose precision.

You mentioned that consumers are generally on a limited budget, and you keep the budget down with MEDLINE, some PDQ, and some Internet thrown in. How do you estimate in advance what the costs will be for a particular search?

For my standard search—which is very simple, to find treatments of a condition—I charge my minimum, about an hour's worth of time. That's a baseline starting point. If it gets more complicated or if I have to go into other sources like alternative medicine, I will give them a range; at that point, I never know how much the extra work is going to cost. Because I search more sources, cancer projects run a bit more—about an hour and a half of time, plus shipping. Usually, though, from the time I start the interview to the time that I print it out and get it in the mail, a simple search takes a good hour.

You mentioned alternative—or what is now being called "complementary"—medicine. How does that fit into your service?

There are several things to say about alternative medicine. One is that there hasn't been a lot of good-quality research done on it, and what has been done has mostly been in Europe, not in the U.S. In the last few years, Congress has mandated funds for more alternative medicine research, and I think we're going to see more quality research coming from that. But right now, I often discourage people who ask for alternative medicine searches. It's not that they shouldn't use alternative medicine, but I have to caution them that whatever information we find is not as credible as what we find in MEDLINE. Right now, the research just isn't the same quality. There would be a great opportunity for a database with good access to good sources.

Where do you go to get information about complementary treatments?

I do some searching on Allied and Complementary Medicine (AMED) [122], through DataStar [154] and Dialog [155]. If I'm desperate, I'll just do a general Web search, but I look everything over very carefully to make sure it's not a commercial for some product or other. If I do find something from a commercial site that I think is good, I will indicate "This is a commercial site," so the client is aware of where it came from.

One of the reasons I shied away from consumer searching, besides the money aspect, was the specter of malpractice. How do you handle it when a client asks, "What do you think I should do?"

I say, "The only thing I can do is get you the research that's out there. I cannot tell you what you have or how to treat it." I have a disclaimer on my brochure and on every search that goes out that says that we're information providers, that this is not intended to be the sole source of their medical information, and that they should consult their own healthcare providers.

Usually, they seem to understand that, even before I do the interview. I have a set of screening questions that are not necessarily formalized, but there are people whom I simply discourage from using the service—like the person who was calling "for a friend."

On a completely different subject, Pam, you've also done market research work for medical device companies. How do consumers differ from the commercial field?

Working with consumers is very limited. The hand-holding is basically confined to the interview. If they have questions, they might call me back, but once the search goes out, that's usually the end of it. With a company, you have to figure out what they want and check with them frequently to make sure you're on track. The end result is different for every project. There's nothing uniform about it.

Another thing is that consumers generally want the results in their hands, and they want them quickly. I usually ship search results within 24 hours of the request. Quite frequently, a person will come back from the doctor and, if the diagnosis is life-threatening, like cancer, they want it right away. If it isn't, they still want it right away, because they're scared. This is a very personal thing.

People who are working in a company setting have a different point of view. They may be on a deadline, they may need it right now, but their lives aren't on the line. Consumers want it in their hands right now. They don't want to have to go any further. I always tell them that we can get articles, but it takes about a week to get them. At least they have the peace of mind of knowing that it's coming.

Another difference with consumers is that not everyone I deal with has a computer, so I print out the reports and send them by express delivery service rather than email. That way, they get it the next day, and it's easier for me to put together a nice presentation that they can follow.

if someone were to say, "I want to go into providing consumer health information," what is the one thing you would tell him or her to do in order to be successful?

The main thing is to have a lot of patience while you grow your business. You must plan on spending probably 80 percent of your time on public relations in the first couple of years. Then you have to keep that effort going. You have to cast a wide net. You cannot target just one particular group or one particular paper. It's almost essential to get national coverage, because not everybody is sick at the moment that your publicity is going out, and you need to reach clients when they need your service. I must admit, though, that I still get calls from people who saw my article in *The Wall Street Journal* back in early 1996. One of the reasons I've been successful in this business is the PR I've done. You cannot just sit in the office and expect the work to come in.

Do you get a lot of repeat business? The perception of consumer health research is that the person gets sick, you get them the information, they get better, and they don't need you anymore.

They don't need you right away, but I have a lot of clients who either have a family member that needs something, too, or they've had a complication. As I mentioned, I also get a lot of clients by word of mouth. Or somebody will cut out something, like the April 1995 *Better Homes and Gardens* article in which I was featured, and save it for years.

You appear to be confident that, if you keep it simple enough and inexpensive enough, you will continue to get consumer business.

Well, I say that now, but it could change. Things are changing very quickly with the Internet and people's access to PubMed and other Internet sites. Many people think they can get it on their own—and they can. They just need to know *what* they're getting. I think a lot of emphasis in the future will be on educating consumers to get it themselves, or educating them that they need an expert to get it for them.

Tell me what an expert brings to the research process that a typical intelligent consumer does not.

Having been involved in one aspect or another of healthcare all my adult life, I am very familiar with the field. I'm very familiar with patients, what they need, and how scared they are. I know that when you're scared, you can't think well or do good work.

I also know medical terminology. If I don't know it, I know how to find it quickly. It's more than just going into the Internet, which a lot of people think is all you need to do. It's having the background, the expertise, the education—having the sympathy, in a way, the compassion to know what people need, why they need it, and how they can get it.

Terminology is a big part of it. You may think you know what your condition is called, but what are the synonyms, what's the clinical phrase, how is it listed in MEDLINE so that you can actually find everything that's relevant in PubMed? That's why I said earlier that you have to be careful about evaluating the research on alternative or complementary medicine, because there isn't a lot of good research out there. Most of it is folklore and what Grandma used to do. That's hard for people to understand.

If someone has a Ph.D. background, they know how to evaluate research. It's a whole art—or a science, really—in itself. How many subjects were involved? What were the conditions? What were the confounding factors? What were the constants? There are all kinds of ways to evaluate whether research is good or not, and that sort of evaluation takes place in MEDLINE, because all those journals are peer-reviewed. But it doesn't usually occur in alternative medicine. You're looking at apples and oranges, because there isn't a standard.

From your consumer health research perspective, what "blue-sky" resource or enhancement would you like to see?

I would like somebody to write all the MEDLINE abstracts in plain English.

Oooh, 8 million MEDLINE abstracts in plain English. I don't think we'll get it.

Well, you said "blue-sky!"

Super Searcher Power Tips

➤ On doing a consumer reference interview

I try to get as much information about them and their condition as I can. I will ask their age. I try to get the exact diagnosis and how it relates to their age and their sex, if there are any complicating factors, anything their doctor has told them that might be relevant. I don't always use all the information, but I like to know as much as I can, so that if I get 500 citations, I can narrow it down a little bit better.

➤ On the doctor as consultant

I coach the consumer client to have a dialogue with the doctor, rather than a confrontation. Doctors can easily be intimidated if you go in and say, "Well, what do you think about this? Why didn't you tell me about this?" I think of a doctor as a consultant. If you ask consultants to help with your business, you pay them a lot of money and they tell you what to do. Then you use your judgment on whether it will work or not for your business. I like to look at doctors that way.

➤ On not giving advice

The only thing I can do is get you the research that's out there. I cannot tell you what you have or how to treat it. I have a disclaimer on my brochure and on every search that goes out that says that we're information providers, that this is not intended to be the sole source of their medical information, and that they should consult their own healthcare providers.

➤ On the need for quick turnaround

Consumers generally want the results in their hands, and they want them quickly. I usually ship within 24 hours. If it's life-threatening, like cancer, they want it right away. If it isn't, they still want it right away, because they're scared. People who are working in a company may be on a deadline; they may need it right now, but their lives aren't on the line.

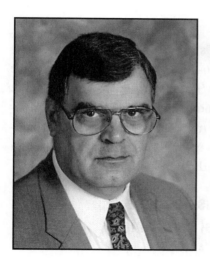

John E. Levis

Independent Healthcare Generalist

John Levis is President of John E. Levis Associates, Inc., a Michigan-based firm providing secondary and primary research in the health and medical industries.

jlevis@ix.netcom.com

John, you have an unusual background for a medical searcher. How did you come to do medical searching?

I've spent 25 years working in and around medicine, beginning as a trained medical photographer at two large hospitals and a medical school. My responsibilities were to provide hospital staff with complete photographic services. That included preparation of lecture slides and photographing X-rays for publication, as well as documenting medical procedures in the operating room or the autopsy room. When I went from a large hospital to a medical school, my responsibilities changed significantly. My staff and I were responsible for providing full audiovisual services for the faculty who trained the medical students. That exposed me to instructional technology, as we were involved in planning the medical training curriculum. Because of that, I became very interested in instructional technology and returned to study it in graduate school.

Somewhat serendipitously, right around that time, the university I was with suffered some pretty significant financial cuts, and I was one of those. While I supported myself with freelance photography work, I came across a book written by Sue Rugge called *The Information Broker's Handbook* [186, see Appendix A]. I began to mull over how I could put together the clinical medical knowledge that I had with my interest in information technology. So, I finally took the plunge and became an independent information professional in medicine.

I know that a large part of your business over the years has been for pharmaceutical companies, attorneys, and some consumers. What kinds of medical questions do you get?

It's very varied. For the attorneys, I do what I call litigation preparation, which is very different from litigation support. Litigation preparation is to help attorneys develop the basic information they need to understand any particular kind of case they may be involved with. As an example of a personal injury case, an individual in an automobile was struck from behind by another automobile and suffered an injury. An MRI was done, nothing was found, yet he was experiencing a great deal of difficulty and pain. Later, he had somehow aggravated the problem, and the subsequent MRI found an injury in his back. The attorney asked me to find the rate of false-negative and/or false-positive MRI injuries, so I did a search of the medical literature and found those rates for him.

Sounds like a "needle-in-a-haystack" search.

Actually, in this case, it was fairly straightforward. I searched MEDLINE [96] and found several articles that gave us the information we needed. In another case, a young man was sprayed by a pesticide, and he suffered a chronic obstructive pulmonary disease type of injury. The medical expert for the opposing side had never physically examined this young man, but rendered an opinion, based on written examinations in the medical records, that this was not a significant injury.

So, the young man's attorney asked me to locate some information to give them an idea of this medical expert's thoughts on the importance of a physical examination. The needle-in-a-haystack reference is rather apt here, because this individual had written a chapter in a book that was a guide for residents coming on to a service. In it, he stated the importance of an actual physical examination before making any determinations. There was only one copy of this book in existence; it was written for one hospital, for one pediatric service, and I was fortunate enough to be able to locate it. As a result, damages were awarded.

How did you ever find out about that book? What was the process you used to uncover it?

The client had supplied me with the medical expert's *curriculum vitae* and the book was listed among his publications. I searched the Detroit Area Library Network's OPAC (Online Public Access Catalog) and didn't find it. I called several area hospital and medical school libraries and was unsuccessful in locating the title. I thought the citation might be incorrect, so I searched MEDLINE for the author of the chapter and for the editor of the book, still with no luck. As a last resort, I contacted a colleague who has a document delivery service, and she located the book on OCLC [168]. A couple of phone calls later, I had a copy of the chapter in hand.

What other types of searches do you do?

I have been asked to locate literature in support of patent applications, for prior art or lack thereof. Those are perhaps less straightforward searches, because they need to be fairly exhaustive, and they often involve searching literature from around the world. I'm asked to do a variety of things for pharmaceutical firms. For example, I was recently asked to locate data on a clinical trial that was conducted outside the United States, and, another time, to uncover chemical structure data on a novel compound. That project required a search of several of the specialized chemical and pharmaceutical files on Dialog [155], as well as a great deal of primary research contacting the appropriate regulatory agencies in the countries involved. Right now, I'm working on an ongoing project for a client who is building a database of new drugs for the treatment of cancer and its related problems.

How do you find those regulatory agencies?

For Europe, EUDRAnet [117] is a great place to start. It's a site run by the European Union, with links to EU regulatory agencies, and then country-by-country links to the medical device and pharmaceutical regulatory agencies of all the member countries. It includes street addresses and telephone numbers, so you can reach them even without an email or Web site address.

In this particular case, I needed Canadian information, so I contacted the Therapeutics Products Programme of Health Canada [121]. By the way, Canada has some very good sites with statistical information.

When a project is that large and extensive, how do you know when you've finished searching?

Very good question. I often ask myself, "Am I finished?" When I'm searching for something like what I've just described, it's a matter of being really exhaustive in the sources that I search. I try to search as many different sources for the information as possible. One is limited, of course, by the budget one's been given, and sometimes that's the deciding factor.

You've given me a great segue. What happens when you think it's going to cost more than your client is willing to spend?

When I start on a large project, I work with the client to establish the budget up front. Sometimes, they have a fairly fixed dollar amount in mind. For a simple literature search, it might only be a few hundred dollars; for a patent literature search, it might be a couple of thousand dollars. But you have to work with the client and establish a budget that covers both time and anticipated cost. If it looks like it's going to require more than that, it's a matter of sitting down with the client and explaining where you're going, where you think you need to go, and asking whether or not they want to go there.

For projects in which you draw on a lot of different resources, what kind of a mix of sources do you use?

For most medical literature searches, there's a standard trinity: MEDLINE, EMBASE [131] and BIOSIS [123]. MEDLINE and EMBASE are very similar in that they are bibliographic. MEDLINE indexes something in the neighborhood of five or six thousand peer-reviewed journals; EMBASE has around 3,500 journals, is more European, and includes more journals devoted to pharmaceutical and pharmacology topics. There's about 30 percent overlap in title coverage; they complement each other very nicely. BIOSIS covers not only journals, but also conference proceedings, books, monographs, and many other sources of literature that you typically don't find in either EMBASE or MEDLINE. So, they make a very good trinity as a starting point.

It then comes down to the kind of information that you're looking for. For instance, if the client is particularly interested in full-text articles, I'll certainly go to Gale's Health and Wellness Database [133]. If we're looking for information that is definitely more pharmaceutically oriented, then I would look at some of the other Dialog files that are cued to pharmaceutical or pharmacologic projects. I do a lot of OneSearches in the Pharmaprojects [145] files; that lets me identify and select the specific files that might hold the data I'm looking for. I also use IMSWorld Product Launches [134] and R&D Focus [135] quite often, along with ADIS Newsletters [43] and ADIS Inpharma [43].

Certainly, the Internet is an important part of any search strategy these days and, depending on the kind of information needed, I would certainly go into some of the Internet sources.

An ongoing pharmaceutical project tracking new cancer compounds involves a lot of searching on the Internet. I look at a number of pharmaceutical and biotech sites such as the online version of the newsletter *Cancer Weekly Plus* [46], the electronic newsletter *Drug Discovery Online* [49], and the news service NewsPage [36]. NewsPage has some wire service coverage, as well as patent applications and more general industry news. It also allows me to build a search and run it when I wish, which in this case is weekly. In some of the other news services, you have to browse headlines each day.

You once said to me that you consider yourself a dinosaur because you still go directly to the National Library of Medicine's ELHILL service to search MEDLINE, and you're planning on holding a wake when it's discontinued. When that happens, where will you search MEDLINE?

Yes, I search MEDLINE directly, although the NLM is apparently going to close down direct access to it later this year. I'm going to burn a candle and say a prayer! I was trained to search MEDLINE directly. There are advantages and disadvantages to any information gateway, and I really like the medical subject headings, the MeSH terminology. MeSH is an extremely well-designed controlled vocabulary, and the direct version allows for great precision. There is a Web-based version—PubMed [112]—that is very popular with end users. PubMeb provides for MeSH searching, too, but not as precisely. You can also use MeSH on the Dialog version of MEDLINE, and I suspect that I will be learning to do that in the not-too-distant future!

It sounds like you're a firm believer in indexing and specialized thesauruses.

There are certainly files in which specialized thesauruses are very useful, and I do use them when they're appropriate to the particular search strategy. I do like controlled vocabularies. They allow me to precisely focus the search strategy. For example, the Gale databases have a business vocabulary that lets you home in on the specific segment of the pharmaceutical market that you're interested in, perhaps the antineoplastic industry or the vaccines industry.

When attorneys ask you to find information because they have a particular case in hand, and you come up with information that completely lays their case to waste, how do you present the results?

I always explain to any attorney whom I work with that the client is theirs, not mine; that I view my responsibility as finding information related to their question, whether it supports the case or not. In some cases, I have found information that is contrary to what the attorney would really like me to find, but that's part of litigation. Their client is not my client. My responsibility is to find good, solid, reliable information; whether or not it supports their side is for them to decide.

How do you format your results?

That's up to the client. In some cases, it's just a matter of rip-and-ship—you find it in the database, pull it out, and send it electronically, as-is. In other cases, I prepare nice-looking word-processed documents or even, occasionally, PowerPoint presentations.

For some reason, the attorneys I work for are always last-minute. It's often a matter of faxing or overnighting photocopies of journal articles. With pharmaceutical companies, the work I do usually ends up in the hands of the market research or competitive intelligence units. Often, that entails putting together a PowerPoint presentation and physically going to the client and presenting the material.

Do you decide which articles to get?

Yes, very often. In some cases, I may present a bibliography including abstracts that the client can choose from. Sometimes, they ask me to pick out two, three, or five that I think are the best. Since much of the information is duplicated from article to article, I sit down and evaluate the content and decide which articles best represent what my client wants to see.

We've mostly talked about your corporate and attorney work. Do you still do research for consumers?

Actually, consumer research has always been one of the more rewarding things I do. Part of the reason I'm not doing as much as I used to is that so much quality information is now available on the Internet. When I first started in business, there was a very serious lack of quality information. Now, with sites like Intelihealth [22], CBSHealthwatch [17], MD Anderson [24], and many more sites from the major medical centers, it's easier for consumers to do their own research.

I think the growth of consumer healthcare sites is very, very important. Health and medical information is way up there on the list of reasons that people access the Internet. There's no doubt that, even five years ago, the quality of medical information was very suspect. One of the first sites I'm familiar with that came online and tried to answer medical questions in a reliable way was Oncolink [26], a site devoted to cancer, which grew out of the old CompuServe Cancer forum. Now, there are many excellent sites for information. All of the major disease associations now have sites that provide excellent information for people.

If a consumer calls and says "I've just been diagnosed with thus and such," are you likely

to do the research, or do you direct them someplace else?

Very often, people are confronted with something that may be devastating news, and they're simply looking for some basic information. Then, I will direct them to an appropriate site. For example, if it's a cancer situation, I will direct them to the National Cancer Institute [98]. The National Cancer Institute has an excellent fax-back service; you can request specific pages of information, and they're faxed to you automatically. I keep the phone number and a list of the order codes for the different documents, and can provide the caller with the specific codes for the information they need. But if people want to use my services, we'll set a maximum budget, and I will research both the Internet and more traditional databases to assemble a fairly comprehensive package that answers their questions.

Do you put a disclaimer on that package?

Yes, I do, and that's a good point. I make sure, in both our initial conversations and my final package, that people understand that I am not a medical professional, and that I am not offering diagnoses. Occasionally, people ask simple things, such as "What's the best hospital?" or "Who's the best doctor?" I am incapable of answering those questions because they're asking for an opinion.

It's good to know that people with access to computers can at least start to find their own information, and if they get into something more intricate, there are people they can call.

Now, the flip side of this is something medical professionals call "Internet Syndrome." People go out and research their illnesses, find the answer they are looking for, then try to convince their physician that that's the best way for them to be treated.

There's actually a medical term called "Internet Syndrome"?

It came up at a medical meeting. Clinicians were complaining and using the term "Internet Syndrome" for people with a disease who were going out, researching information, and finding treatments that they thought they needed to have. Then, the physician has to spend time explaining why that particular treatment isn't applicable in their particular case. So, yes, there is a medical term called "Internet Syndrome."

With all the new resources out there for professional researchers, how do you keep up?

I read a fair amount of industry literature. I subscribe to *Online* magazine [64], *EContent* [51], *Searcher* [68], and *Information Today* [56], and I try to read as much as I can. I'm active in a couple of professional associations, the Association of Independent Information Professionals [75] and the Society of Competitive Intelligence Professionals [79]. Both produce journals, but, more importantly, they give you an opportunity to network about sources with colleagues and peers.

For medical sources, I subscribe to several newsgroups like sci.med, sci.med.bio, sci.med.pharmacy, and harvard.sci.review, and some general news portals, such as NewsPage. I subscribe to *Genetic Engineering News* [54], which is a newspaper-type publication that helps me keep up. It's extremely difficult to stay abreast. We're inundated with data, but it's becoming harder and harder to mine the information out of it.

How do you evaluate information you find online?

Certainly, in terms of medical searching, it's extremely important that the information you obtain comes from credible sources. For that reason, I search primarily in the more trusted sources like MEDLINE or EMBASE or BIOSIS—sources in which there's been at least a first cut at assuring the reliability of information. Peer review is important, and that's another reason why I tend to go to the Dialog or Dow Jones [156] types of services, as opposed to the Internet.

Do you ever just do a general search on the Web?

Oh, absolutely! If it's a new device or something that hasn't been written about much in the peer-reviewed literature, very often I will just throw a few terms into a search engine to see what happens. Then I sit down, get the 2,300,000 hits, and go through them very quickly to get some background on the subject before I even begin to think about how I want to really search for it.

I do something similar using Dialindex in Dialog, trying to identify sources with some information about the topic, and simply learning the language that attaches itself to that new procedure or device. I've had medical experts ask for information about a particular device using jargon they're very familiar and comfortable with. Unfortunately, the jargon turns out not to be the way the industry refers to the product. It's not as unusual as one might think to find out that the terminology one is using is not appropriate to the search.

What do you look for in a general search engine?

Actually, I don't look for anything in particular, because none of the search engines out there do a very good job of searching the Internet. The general search engines, such as HotBot [150], Lycos [152], or Yahoo! [153], don't discriminate between sites that offer unproven treatments or non-reviewed literature and the sites from more credible sources. I use two or three or four of them and hope that I get a fairly good representation of what's out there.

Occasionally, I use a medical search engine, such as HealthAtoZ [21] or Medical World Search [9]. One of the nice things about these sites is that they restrict themselves to health information only. At least the information is filtered, even if only slightly, through a peer-review process. You're more likely to avoid the unproven information that you get when you try to search for medical information using the general search engines. I also tend to stick to sites that I know fairly well, simply because a lot of what I do is in a tight time frame. Since I charge for my time, I don't want to sit around just fishing. Even on the Internet, I tend to stick to more traditional sources.

If somebody created the ideal research resource for you, what might it look like?

I can speculate that there probably is no such thing for me, simply because the kinds of things that I'm looking for vary so much from day to day.

Super Searcher Power Tips

➤ On budgeting the project

I work with the client to establish the budget up front. For a simple literature search, it might only be a few hundred dollars; for a patent literature search, it might be a couple of thousand dollars. But you have to work with the client and establish a budget that covers both time and anticipated cost. If it looks like it's going to require more than that, it's a matter of sitting down and explaining where you're going, where you think you need to go, and asking whether or not they want to go there.

➤ On working with attorneys

I always explain that the client is theirs, not mine; that I view my responsibility as finding information related to their question, whether it supports their case or not. In some cases, I have found information that is contrary to what the attorneys would really like me to find, but that's part of litigation. Their client is not my client. My responsibility is to find good, solid, reliable information; whether or not it supports their side is for them to decide.

➤ On formatting search results

That's really up to the client. In some cases, it's just a matter of rip-and-ship—find it in the database, pull it out, and send it electronically, as-is. Sometimes, I prepare nice-looking word-processed documents. For some reason, the attorneys I work for are always last-minute. It's often a matter of faxing or overnighting photocopies of journal articles. With pharmaceutical companies, it might entail putting together a PowerPoint presentation and physically going to the client and presenting the material.

➤ On learning new terminology

If it's a new device or something that hasn't been written about much in the peer-reviewed literature, very often I will just throw a few terms into a general search engine to see what happens. Then I sit down, get the 2,300,000 hits, and go through them very quickly to get some background on the subject before I even begin to think about how I want to really search for it. I do the same thing using Dialindex in Dialog, trying to identify sources with some information about the topic and simply learning the language that attaches itself to that new procedure or device.

➤ On finding regulatory agencies

For Europe, EUDRAnet is a great place to start. It's a site run by the European Union, with links to EU regulatory agencies, and then country-by-country links to the medical device and pharmaceutical regulatory agencies of all the member countries. It includes street addresses and telephone numbers, so you can reach them even without an email or Web site address.

➤ On using a specialized thesaurus

There are certainly files in which specialized thesauruses are very useful, and I do use them when they're appropriate to the particular search strategy. I do like controlled vocabularies. They allow me to precisely focus the search strategy. For example, the Gale databases have a business vocabulary that lets you home in on the specific segment of the pharmaceutical market that you're interested in.

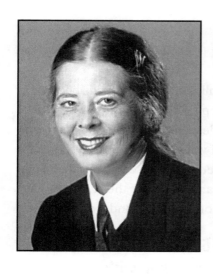

Bonnie Snow

Following Pharmaceuticals

Bonnie Snow, MLS, is Director of Client Services for the eKnowledge Group, part of Caredata.com, Inc., an online syndicator of healthcare content.

bonnie.snow@caredata.com
snow@citizen1.com

Bonnie, your name is synonymous in many searchers' minds with writing about online health and medical information. How did you come to be so immersed in this field?

I think I'm just lucky. My undergraduate degree was in English literature. I tried a number of different jobs, including public school teaching, before I decided to go into librarianship. When I completed my graduate degree, I went to work at the Philadelphia College of Pharmacy and Science, a major resource library with a great deal of funding and an outstanding collection. The College had established a tradition of providing *carte blanche* information services to their pharmacist alumni on the phone, and that immediately plunged me into the library's reference collection, which was outstanding. I got to know a lot about it.

That was the dawn of online, of course, when it was only MEDLARS. It was a wonderful environment. Before I left the College, I was beginning to teach accredited courses and do bibliographic instruction as well. I'd also done quite a bit of writing and was encouraged to submit articles for publication.

Then, going to work for Dialog [155, see Appendix A] gave me unlimited online time.

Medical information is a really worthwhile field, because it does affect the quality of people's lives. I continue to write because I enjoy it, and there's a desperate need for information in the medical area. I found that I write as much for myself as for anyone else, to get down on paper whatever search problem I had worked on, really delve into it, and get it out there. Then I have something to refer to in helping other people find it on their own.

You now work for Caredata.com [160], which consolidates its own syndicated information with healthcare industry data from a number of different sources and makes it available to subscribers. What's your role there?

I'm the Director of Client Services for their eKnowledge division, which means that I am in charge of instruction in our own software. I also help clients formulate ways to find information from our sources and, if necessary, from other databases. I am in charge of the teaching function. I develop the training material, hard-copy and online user aids, and do some teaching myself. I'm also responsible for outreach to the information workers' community. That includes not just the traditional information professional, but also knowledge workers—that is, market researchers and the like, who might not have a background in professional information retrieval, but who have become the new intermediaries.

In addition, I see that you teach a class on searching for information about alternative medicine.

Yes. I teach for the Medical Library Association [77], which has a rigorous and ongoing continuing education and accreditation process. It began with a course in drug and pharmaceutical

resources. Over the years, I've developed courses in many different areas. They asked me to develop the alternative medicine
course in 1994, and it has turned out to be a real favorite. Many of
the people who participate in that course are hospital librarians.
There is a rising urgency on the part of the medical profession to
know more about alternative medicine, because consumers are
being exposed to it so much more. The Web is driving some of
that exposure, as is increased consumer activism in the healthcare area. So, librarians are looking to build their knowledge base.
I've had people take the course more than once, because it's a
moving target; I revise it about every six months.

I saw a quote from CNN [34] that "Americans who try alternative medicine generally use it to supplement, not replace, more usual U.S. methods of healthcare." Are you finding that true on the searching end also?

Yes. That's why "alternative" is not really as accurate as "complementary," which is more the European terminology. Our own
government agency, which used to be the Office of Alternative
Medicine, is now the National Center for Complementary and
Alternative Medicine [99]. It's common sense. In our society, if
you are a user of physician services, you're more likely to also be
a user of alternative therapies. That's different from many other
countries, since you are likely to rely more on folk medicine in
Third World countries.

I would not use the term "traditional medicine," because "traditional" in the establishment medicine context means folk
medicine. I tend to call it "mainstream medicine." When you
look at the complementary medicine literature, sometimes they
contrast what they are doing with "traditional." But if you use
"traditional" in MEDLINE, you're going to get traditional
Chinese medicine. That's one of the things I love about searching—our language is very unpredictable.

What would a typical question be that would lead you to use both mainstream and complementary sources?

Actually, I would have to get a cue that someone was interested in the complementary sources. People usually know whether they are or not. Much more typically, I run into someone who simply says, "I need to know the possible complementary modalities that we need to be aware of that might cause interaction problems with the mainstream therapies." Very rarely would I automatically get both, but, depending on the requestor, I would be more inclined now to ask if that was an area of concern. We know that people don't always ask everything on their agenda without some prompting. That's part of the process, of course, getting as much as you can out of the requestor before you go on.

It sounds like a variation on the reference interview.

Yes. The interview is about finding out what people need and encouraging them to tell you more, to tell the story, as it were. People rarely ask what they really need to know, so finding out their context is extremely important. With end users, I often have to get back to them after I explore the topic area and say, "I'm finding this; is this something that you need?" So, I have to leave that door open.

I think all searching is iterative, or it's probably not very good. You find something, you do a reality check, and then you're not afraid to go back to the beginning to look for more, based on what you found. That's one of the ways to use the Web; there's so much free out there that you can do a lot of preliminary checking to get some of the vocabulary and so on before you tackle the big, expensive files.

What files would you normally use for a mainstream search?

I consider there to be a "big four" in medicine: MEDLINE [96], EMBASE [131], BIOSIS Previews [123] and SciSearch [147] are baseline for me. Then, I go on to the specialty files that would complement that subject area. But I always try to get enough budget or leeway to look at SciSearch because of its multidisciplinary approach, the cover-to-cover indexing, the cited-reference capabilities, and the incredible timeliness. I almost always find that it fills in some blanks that the others are not picking up.

I get very frustrated because budgetary constraints, or just overall skepticism, sometimes keep people from SciSearch. People are frightened by it, I think, because it is a bit more expensive, and because it's entirely natural language. It's not indexed by human beings, and it's not a controlled vocabulary, so you have to think of lots of synonyms. Of course, we face that whenever we go into full-text files. That's the wonderful thing about what's happening with information—there's lots more full text. But it also means vocabulary, vocabulary, vocabulary.

I'm sometimes concerned that so much is available in full text that people tend to go for the easy shot. They don't go on to use the bibliographic files to find articles that aren't available in full text online, although that would have been exactly what they needed.

Yes. I think that's a major concern. That's particularly important in medicine, because they may have missed something that could really affect the patient-care situation or the business decision. End users in particular tend to think, "Well, I've gotten this, and this must be all there is," not realizing at all that there's tons more and that they really need to look at those other sources. I absolutely agree that it's frightening.

I think evidence-based medicine is also encouraging this; people are taught to evaluate a clinical study and look for outcomes research. Instead of starting broad and then narrowing down, they start narrow. Then, because starting narrow takes a lot of work, they never go on to a broader search.

Can I ask you to define "evidence-based medicine"?

It's medicine based on scientific data that can be replicated. The gold standard is the double-blind study: Look at the evidence that's available, evaluate those studies, pool that evidence by meta-analysis and, especially, look for that randomized controlled trial. Students at medical and pharmacy schools are getting heavily into EBM and outcomes research and on learning to evaluate a study. I think it's wonderful that people are being taught to evaluate the literature and not just assume that all clinical studies are equally rigorous. However, they pride themselves so much on being able to analyze a clinical study and look for its flaws and key points, that it tends to narrow their focus. They don't consider the other things that one needs to take into account in answering a question. If you only look at certain journals, such as *JAMA* [55] and *British Medical Journal* [45] and *Annals of Internal Medicine* [44], you miss many other peer-reviewed articles to which the bibliographic databases alert you. The major advantage of automated current-awareness services is to broaden your horizons, to get good current contents from a whole spectrum of sources. I think one of our jobs is to get those students hooked on those current-awareness services.

Any particular current-awareness services you'd recommend?

No, anything that will give them what they need. All the traditional online services have a means whereby you can customize output using the keywords you're looking for. Again, I'm a big advocate of making sure something as timely as SciSearch is included. I'm also a big advocate of looking at the industry newsletters, such as *Scrip* [67] and *The Pink Sheet* [69], because they can distill so much and bring in business and regulatory aspects that affect healthcare. I don't know anywhere else you can find some of that information.

I've started using several of the news tracker services on various Web portals. I would miss so much if I limited it to just one. Each one has different tracking capabilities; some allow proximity searching, some offer "must have" term searching versus "should have."

I looked at some of those to augment what I was already getting in the fee-based services. I was dissatisfied with a lot of the free sources, though, because they don't specifically target healthcare industry professionals. But I agree with you; you always have to look at more than one source. I go into a lot of the better journal sites and sign up for a free email alert on their entire table of contents. WebMedLit [16], for example, monitors 22 or 23 journals for you. It lets you choose a plain table of contents current-awareness service or one filtered by keyword.

I'm not that concerned about filtering, because I don't know what I want until I see it. For example, in product development, we need to look for trends and hot topics so we can predict what information people will be needing. When a topic is fairly new, you can't express it with just a few keywords. That's part of its newness—the language hasn't gelled. So I need to just browse and browse and browse.

Earlier in the conversation, you said that, when you're doing a search, you'd go to the "big four" and then add the specialty files. Which

specialty files would you be looking at and for which subjects?

I try to make sure that an online service provides the full repertoire. For example, International Pharmaceutical Abstracts [138] is a gem of a database for specialized clinical topics. I wouldn't consult it for standard kinds of clinical questions, because it's not very timely. However, for herbal or pharmacy practice questions, or nitty-gritty questions, such as the effect of dosage form on efficacy, that's where International Pharmaceutical Abstracts really shines. It indexes some unique journals. It's excellent in alternative medicine and particularly the herbal area, because pharmacognosy, the study of naturally-derived drugs, is a pharmacy school degree. It's a small file; it never really competes in terms of numbers of references when lined up with the others, but the quality of those references is outstanding. Other than EMBASE, it's the only medical file that indexes brand names in a special field.

Then, of course, there are a lot of specialty databases that I call the "pipeline directories." Some of my favorites are IMSWorld R&D Focus [135], Pharmaprojects [145], ADIS R&D Insight [43], NME Express (New Molecular Entity Express) [144], Drugs of the Future [50], and Drug Data Report [48]. Also, NDA Pipeline [60], although that focuses more on the U.S. pipeline. Those are the files that look at what's in the pharmaceutical pipeline, pre-clinical to post-launch. Each, in its own way, enables you to get at what stage the drug is in. Some of the better ones provide some bibliography or patent information; a few let you examine a pharmacological class and all the therapeutic applications being investigated. They tend to be quite expensive files, but they are very valuable. A lot of the joy I had in working with Dialog was that a big part of my job was teaching people the significant differences among these databases and how to use them together.

I've been asked, "Why bother going to Pharmaprojects, now that the Pharmaceutical

Research and Manufacturers of America (PhRMA) [78] has a drugs-in-development database online?" How would you answer that?

I have to laugh, as you probably do, too. Anyone who does even one sample search on a given topic in the two databases is going to see a dramatic difference in results. It is immediately apparent that PhRMA's is a very selective database. They solicit input from their membership and, hopefully, look at a few other sources, but I suspect it's best with their membership's products.

Publishing companies, such as PJB, ADIS, and IMSWorld, pursue many different avenues to get the information they have. They check it with the company but, unless there's an outright denial of the information they've uncovered, they put it online. They check news sources, regularly attend investment meetings, look at market research reports, go to scientific meetings, and do everything they can to find out more. They also have some leverage because, if a company is covered in the pipeline databases, that boosts its Wall Street ratings.

The commercial entities are much more proactive in assembling information from a variety of sources and keeping it up-to-date. To get good pipeline information, you have to pay for it. It costs them a lot to produce these files, and I think that's why they are so expensive. But, on the other hand, if you are in the pharmaceutical industry and don't have that kind of competitive intelligence, you're probably not going to be in the industry for very long.

A lot of people tell me they can't afford to search all of the pipelines, and they ask me, "If you had to pick, which would be the one?" Of course, there isn't just one, because some are better for certain questions than others. In most cases, I've been able to help people prepare a proposal to get at least two or three out of the six or seven databases that are out there.

What tricks would you suggest in order to get the most out of those expensive databases? There must be ways to minimize your exposure.

Often, there aren't, to tell you the truth. They're purposely constructed so that a sound bite isn't enough. I think the best defense is to really have studied those databases and figured out their differences. I've prepared an awful lot of charts where I list "If I need to search by therapeutic class …," "If I need to search by pharmacology …," "If I need to search by company, licensee, phase of development …," and so on. There's a standard list of data points that people need to check in the pipeline and need to combine in their searches.

Then, I'll cross-tabulate and figure out which files are best for which purpose. Not everyone spends enough time in the files to be totally familiar with them, so I'd just make sure I have those charts ready. It's the information professional's responsibility to be prepared, that is, to construct or assemble user aids, or demand those aids from vendors. The big vendors still have subject specialists, who are very proactive in keeping up and who will often be able to provide you with user aids that clarify the files and indicate how best to search them.

Then there are people like yourself who are writing for industry journals and building comparison charts.

Yes, and those constantly need updating. I think we need more of that. One of my pet peeves is that people are not being evaluative enough. There are wonderful subject hubs that have done a good job of being a vacuum cleaner for the Web, but they hardly ever give any substantive evaluative commentary. It's as if they're afraid they're going to be sued. I get so annoyed that the only comments you find are glowing or nothing at all. Evaluation is a natural part of our job, and it's even more critical now because there's so much more stuff out there!

During the course of this conversation, you've spoken both highly and negatively about the Web. What place does the Web have in a medical researcher's toolkit?

That's a tough one. I'd say, overall, it's a good starting place for vocabulary, which is the difference between success and failure in a search. If you don't have the vocabulary and the appropriate keywords beyond what the requestor thinks are the right ones, you're not going to be able to do a good job. The Web is a good place to find out more about the topic, what the technology is, who's involved in it, and to get some of the terminology.

The Web is a key source in the epidemiological and statistical area. I think it's better than traditional online in that respect. That is one area in which the governments of the world are doing a good job. The Web is also, obviously, a place to monitor the popular pulse, find out what consumers are saying about your product, and be alerted—whether it's completely false or not— that there might be a problem with a perceived adverse effect or interaction. I advise companies to look at the Web for that purpose. Many alternative medicine sites have their own little newsletters that are almost the equivalent of an online chat. They don't have a widespread circulation, but you see what's being said and what people are interested in.

The Web, of course, is also a place to look for some full-text journals. For example, I looked at the *New England Journal of Medicine* [61] site and found that some of their articles are free— some that I had already paid a commercial vendor for. The journals are making an incredible amount available for free. I read recently that someone used Northern Light's Special Collection [157] to search because it has more power than the search engines at individual publication sites, but then went on to print out full-text articles from free sources found elsewhere on the Web.

Obviously, the Internet is a wonderful source for information from organizations—pamphlets and so on that used to be called "vertical file" material. The Web is *the* place to look for calendars of forthcoming events—medical school curricula, conferences, seminars, that kind of thing. And it's obviously the first place to stop for news, now that networks like CNN and MSNBC [35] are covering medical news a bit more.

How do you keep up with all the new sources that are out there?

I don't feel I can ever really keep up with it all. I focus on keeping up in my subject area, that is, pharmaceutical regulatory and corporate developments, new areas in which products are being developed, that kind of thing. There's a real business twist to medicine when you're dealing with it in the corporate world; it is not strictly a clinical thing. Sometimes I'm alerted to new resources through things like *Scrip*; PJB has a wonderful section on their Web site called Pharmapages, devoted to Internet issues in the healthcare industry. I also look at *HMS Beagle*, which is produced by BioMedNet [1], to note what their discussions are focusing on. I'm fortunate that I work for a company whose whole job is to find information sources, organize them, annotate them, and get them out there in our software. I love it when a client asks me to help with something; it gives me a perfect excuse to go out there and wallow in it.

I look at publications like *Online* [64], *EContent* [51], and *Information Today* [56], but frankly, they often pile up on my desk until something arises that prompts me to look back at the professional literature. Once a month, I'll spend a day indulging myself in just looking at information professional literature. Of course, I also hear about new developments at conferences and talks, or just networking at meetings, browsing around an exhibit area, and hearing from customers.

Do you subscribe to any mailing lists?

The only one I participate in is the SLA Pharmaceutical Division's discussion list [175]. I belonged to a few others for awhile, but I unsubscribed because life is short, and I found that it wasn't a good investment of my time. Maybe I just haven't hit the right one.

What happens when you can't find something you're looking for? What's your next step?

Very rarely can you not find anything, particularly now with the Web. It just means thinking up a different approach. Sometimes, you have to step back and go a little bit broader. For example, I had a question in the healthcare statistical area. That's a fascinating and wonderful area, but it can be incredibly difficult. We were looking for statistics on the use of a particular surgical procedure, and needed to get it down to a country-by-country level. We talked about associations and visited the sites of companies that market products used in that procedure. It's amazing how often company home pages provide large amounts of market research data, because they're talking to their stockholders.

Then we discussed looking at investment analyst reports and industry reports. The budget allowed us to go into databases like Investext [139], which is one of my favorite sources for market research statistics. I like sources that have some commentary attached, because they give me a feel for the market. Many of the investment analyst and market research reports can fulfill the function of a mentor for market researchers as well as information professionals. You can very quickly get a snapshot of an industry from a good report.

It sounds like you help end users as well as intermediaries.

That's part of my role at Caredata.com. I think my favorite people to help are, indeed, end users. I really like clinicians and scientists, but market researchers have become much more savvy on the clinical side, and try to keep up on both. That's quite an achievement. They're much more open and inquiring than they used to be, and don't have budgetary constraints, which is wonderful. Time- and attention-span constraints, yes, but the people who have to prepare the reports still recognize that they need to cover all the bases.

Since you teach a class on alternative medicine resources, can you give me an idea of the differences between searching for complementary medicine versus mainstream medicine?

There's not a lot of codified literature out there, even though we've come a long way since the publication of the first Eisenberg study [180] in the early 1990s. Back then, David Eisenberg and a team of researchers at Beth Israel Deaconess Medical Center in Boston found that almost 34 percent of Americans use some kind of complementary medicine. Eisenberg's two major surveys are probably the benchmark of how pervasive complementary medicine is, at least until the government releases cumulative results from the National Health Interview Survey [101], since they added more questions about alternative medicine.

The Eisenberg studies were a wake-up call for the medical profession, after which we began to see alternative medicine being integrated as an elective into medical school curricula. Public consciousness began rising as the media latched onto it, and a lot of feature articles have appeared in major magazines and newspapers. Then, the Dietary Supplement Health and Education Act of 1994 [179] legitimized and regularized some of the product labeling. The *U.S. Pharmacopeia* [170] is also beginning to make herbal monographs available.

So, we're beginning to build a body of evidence to look at, but much of the legitimate research began only in the past decade. In the complementary medicine area, it is more difficult for people to judge what constitutes authority. It can be difficult even for information professionals. You have to look at the studies themselves and also at the kinds of references they cite when published.

Secondly, the Web plays a much more major role as a resource in the complementary medicine area than do the traditional fee-based systems. But again, to collect actual evidence that would be acceptable in the clinical and research world, one couldn't rely, for the most part, on what's out there on the Web.

How do you know what terms to use in a search when the body of literature hasn't been codified?

That *is* one of the challenges. It's not just that there isn't an established canon; even getting the vocabulary is difficult. The more you talk about something, the more it becomes standardized. Some aspects of alternative medicine are so new that the terminology is all over the map. It's fun, I think, to tackle that problem of building your vocabulary in a new area. Sometimes you have to go all over the place to figure out what these people are talking about. You can't just trot to a medical dictionary and find out. At the base of all of online searching is vocabulary. It's the key. It's just more difficult in this area.

Another difference between searching complementary versus mainstream medicine is that it is more difficult for people to be dispassionate about the subject. This creates a bit of a problem. When I first started teaching the MLA course in 1994, there was a healthy skepticism that was almost adversarial about what they, the course participants, were finding. Now, I'm seeing almost the opposite—that people have become advocates. Mainstream medicine has such a broad spectrum of topics that you don't have personal experience with every disease and drug that you're asked to research. With complementary medicine, the people who are searching are among the potential users of the information. People are so desperate for information that it's possible to perhaps accept something of lower quality without giving the usual warnings to your clients.

I have some concern about that; we searchers need to work on that dispassion and objective judgment. Someone attending the course even cited the 1938 Food, Drug and Cosmetic Act as part of the reason why people were using alternatives. They said the Food and Drug Administration [89] was restricting so much of what was available that they forced a lot of the good therapies underground. I was very taken aback by that. Our current drug law has protected our safety and is the model for the entire world's drug laws. To attribute some of the current rise of interest in alternative medicine to that law seems a bit extreme.

Is the government ever a source of information for complementary medicine?

Yes, there's the National Center for Complementary and Alternative Medicine [99] site, which has the CAM (Complementary and Alternative Medicine) Citation Index [86], a subset of MEDLINE. The Office of Dietary Supplements [108] has its own site, with the IBIDS [94] database, in the dietary supplement area. It does tend to be very botanically and horticulturally oriented. Some of the commercial providers have picked up *U.S. Pharmacopeia* herbal and vitamin monographs and mounted them on their free sites, so they're embedded in other sources.

What about commercial databases, such as Allied and Complementary Medicine [122]?

That comes out of the U.K.; for years it was only available on DataStar [154]. Now, it's available through several vendors, but I understand that the funding behind it is poor. They index only about 350 journals, but they cover some very nice homeopathy sources that aren't picked up elsewhere. MANTIS, Manual Alternative and Natural Therapy [141], is also on several commercial vendors. Under its old title, CHIROLARS, it focused very much on the chiropractic area, but it's expanded its scope. Another one is NAPRALERT [143], the Natural Products Alert database from the University of Illinois, on STN [159]. NAPRALERT is very much a pharmacognosy database, very biochemically oriented.

There are some very good complementary medicine resources out there, but there's also some really bad stuff, and distinguishing among them takes some homework. I tell people to sit down and spend some time getting familiar with what's available. If you just wait until the question arises and then use some general search engine, you're dead in the water.

After all we've discussed, where is online searching going?

I don't know. Anyone who's lived in my lifetime has already seen such dramatic changes that, if anything, it's taught us that the sky's the limit. Whenever the old guard begins talking, we all mention our first PC. I remember having to use punched cards to access mainframe computers in graduate school; PCs didn't exist. The revolution in our profession was the personal computer, and the difference it made in terms of access.

Obviously, the World Wide Web also truly revolutionized the information world, and that will continue. Who knows where that is going? The capabilities are just astonishing—the ability to have images; hypertext linkage that mimics thought patterns and encourages less hierarchical thinking. The way that technology has been implemented is just so amazing, I still have revelation moments when I say, "Whoa! I can't believe this! Isn't this incredible?"

But as we get access to more and more information, the need will increase, I think, for more quality filtering. We have challenges ahead of us—in establishing authority, protection from misinformation, and ethical issues. Basically, the Web is uncontrolled. There's an awful lot out there that is dangerous; but, at the same time, we have to be careful about freedom of speech. I don't know how that will all shake out. I think we're going to rely more and more on subject specialty engines, and on human input in addition to machine input, to make some qualitative judgments.

That sounds like a segue into what searchers will have to be able to do in the future.

Yes. And you know, I don't think it's any different from what they've had to do all along. I think they will still have to be very verbal people who know and enjoy language and know the way it works—our language as well as others; obviously, Latin and

Greek word roots are important in medicine. Good preparation for being a searcher is to play a lot of word games, Scrabble and so on. Obviously, logic is also important. An eager and inquiring mind, a person who is a vacuum cleaner, one who will go out there and do widespread reading and exploration, one who enjoys facts and stores them away.

Past work in general reference librarianship and a liberal arts education have served me well. I think it's important not to specialize too much at the outset. At the same time, there is simply too much out there in the medical area and the sciences for everyone to be able to do everything equally well. So, it's the equivalent of the holistic approach in medicine—know a bit about everything but develop knowledge and analytical skills in some specialty areas in order to be genuinely good at evaluating resources.

Super Searcher Power Tips

➤ On searching for alternative therapies

I would not use the term "traditional medicine," because "traditional" in the establishment medicine context means folk medicine. I tend to call it "mainstream medicine." When you look in the complementary medicine literature, sometimes they will contrast what they are doing with "traditional." But if you use "traditional" in MEDLINE, you're going to get traditional Chinese medicine.

➤ On the iterative reference interview

People rarely ask what they really need to know, so finding out their context is extremely important. With end users, I often have to get back to them after I explore the topic area and say, "I'm finding this; is this something that you need?" I have to leave that door open. I think all of searching is iterative, or it's probably not very good. You find something, you do a reality check, and then you're not afraid to go back to the beginning to look for more, based on what you found.

➤ On the importance of SciSearch

I always try to get people to look at SciSearch because of its multidisciplinary approach, the cover-to-cover indexing, the cited reference capabilities, and the incredible timeliness. I've almost always found that it fills in some blanks that the others are not picking up. People are frightened by it, I think, because it is a bit more expensive, and because it's entirely natural language.

➤ On expanding beyond evidence-based medicine

It's wonderful that people are being taught to evaluate the literature and not just assume that all clinical studies are equally rigorous. However, they pride themselves so much on being able to analyze a clinical study and look for its flaws and key points, that it tends to narrow their focus. If you only look at certain journals, like *JAMA*, *British Medical Journal*, and *Annals of Internal Medicine*, you miss many other peer-reviewed articles that bibliographic databases alert you to.

➤ On keeping up with developments in medicine

I was dissatisfied with a lot of the free sources, because they don't specifically target healthcare industry professionals. So, I go into a lot of the better journal sites and sign up for a free email alert on their entire tables of contents. WebMedLit, for example, monitors 22 or 23 journals for you. It lets you choose a plain table of contents current-awareness service or one filtered by keyword.

➤ On finding new drugs before they're launched

There are a lot of specialty databases that I call the "pipeline" directories. Those are the files that look at what's in the pharmaceutical pipeline, pre-clinical to post-launch. Each, in its own way, enables you to get at what stage the drug is in. To get good pipeline information, you have to pay for it. It costs a lot to produce these files, and I think that's why they are so expensive. But, on the other hand, if you are in the pharmaceutical industry and don't have that kind of competitive intelligence, you're probably not going to be in the industry for very long.

➤ On using the Web

The Web is a good starting place for vocabulary, which is the difference between success and failure in a search. If you don't have the vocabulary and the appropriate keywords beyond what the requestor thinks are the right ones, you're not going to be able to do a good job. It's a good place to find out more about the topic, the technology, who's involved in it, and to get some of the terminology.

➤On learning about a new market

I like sources like Investext that have some commentary attached, because they give me a feel for the market. I think many investment analyst and market research reports can fulfill the function of a mentor for market researchers as well as information professionals. You can very quickly get a snapshot of an industry from a good report.

➤ On searching for complementary medicine

In alternative medicine, one has to look at the studies themselves and also at the kinds of references they cite. The Web plays a much more major role as a resource in the complementary medicine area than do the traditional fee-based systems. But to collect actual evidence that would be acceptable in the clinical and research world, one can't rely, for the most part, on the Web. I always tell people to spend some time familiarizing themselves with the good alternative medicine databases that are available. If you just wait until the question arises, and then use some general search engine, you're dead in the water.

Appendix A:

Internet Resources

MEDICAL SITES AND SEARCH ENGINES

1. **BioMedNet**
   www.bmn.com

2. **Hardin MD**
   www.lib.uiowa.edu/hardin/md

3. **Healthfinder**
   www.healthfinder.gov

4. **HealthWeb**
   healthweb.org

5. *JAMA* **NetSight**
   www.medsitenavigator.com/features/Jama

6. **MD Consult**
   www.mdconsult.com

7. **MedHunt**
   www.hon.ch

8. **Medical Matrix**
   www.medmatrix.org

9. **Medical World Search**
   www.mwsearch.com

10. **Medscape**
    www.medscape.com

11. **MedWeb**
    www.medweb.emory.edu/medweb/default.htm

12. **Megasite Project**
    www.lib.umich.edu/megasite

13. **Nursing & Health Care Resources on the Net**
    www.shef.ac.uk/~nhcon

14. **The Virtual Hospital**
    www.vh.org

15. **Web Sites for Internists**
    www.acponline.org

16. **WebMedLit**
    www.webmedlit.com

CONSUMER HEALTH AND MEDICAL SITES

17. **CBSHealthwatch**
    www.cbshealthwatch.com

18. **DrKoop.com**
    www.drkoop.com

19. **Family Village**
    www.familyvillage.wisc.edu

20. **familydoctor.org**
    www.familydoctor.org

21. **HealthAtoZ**
    www.HealthAtoZ.com

22. **InteliHealth**
    www.intelihealth.com

23. **Mayo Clinic Health Oasis**
    www.mayohealth.org

24. **MD Anderson**
    www.mdanderson.org

25. **NOAH (New York Online Access for Health)**
    www.noah.cuny.edu

26. **Oncolink**
    cancer.med.upenn.edu

27. **Onhealth**
    www.onhealth.com

28. **Quackwatch**
    www.quackwatch.com

29. **REPRORISK**
    www.micromedex.com/products/pd-reprorisk.htm

30. **Self-Help Sourcebook Online**
    mentalhelp.net/selfhelp

31. **ThriveOnline**
    www.thriveonline.com

32. **WebMD**
    my.webmd.com

CURRENT MEDICAL NEWS

33. **1stHeadlines-Health**
    www.1stheadlines.com/health1.htm

34. **CNN**
    cnn.com/HEALTH

35. **MSNBC**
    www.msnbc.com/news/HEALTH_Front.asp?ta=y

36. **NewsPage**
    www.individual.com/browse/industry.shtml?level1=46610

REFERENCE BOOKS ONLINE

37. *The Directory of Medical Specialists*
    www.certifieddoctor.org

38. **emedicine.com**
    emedicine.com

39. *Harrison's Online*
    www.harrisonsonline.com

40. *Iowa Family Practice Handbook*
    www.vh.org/Providers/ClinRef/FPHandbook/FPContents.html

41. **STAT!Ref**
    statref.tetondata.com

JOURNALS AND NEWSLETTERS
(Note: Some of these periodicals are available in print as well as online.)

42. *ACP Journal Club*
    www.acponline.org/index.html

43. **ADIS Inpharma; ADIS Newsletters; ADIS R&D Insight**
    www.adis.com

44. *Annals of Internal Medicine*
    www.acponline.org/journals/annals/annaltoc.htm

45. *British Medical Journal*
    www.bmj.com

46. *Cancer Weekly Plus*
    www.newsrx.com

47. *Consumer Reports on Health*
    www.consumerreports.org/Services/health.html

48. **Drug Data Report**
    www.prous.es/product/journal/ddr.html

49. *Drug Discovery Online*
    www.drugdiscoveryonline.com

50. **Drugs of the Future**
    www.prous.es/product/journal/dof.html

51. *EContent*
    www.ecmag.net

52. *Evidence-Based Medicine*
    www.acponline.org/catalog/journals/ebm.htm

53. **F-D-C Reports**
    www.fdcreports.com

54. **Genetic Engineering News**
    www.genwire.com

55. *JAMA—Journal of the American Medical Association*
    jama.ama-assn.org

56. *Information Today*
    www.infotoday.com/it/itnew.htm

57. **MD Computing**
    www.mdcomputing.com

58. *The Medical Letter on Drugs and Therapeutics*
    www.medletter.com

59. *Medicine on the Net*
    www.mednet-i.com

60. **NDA Pipeline**
    www.ndapipeline.com

61. *New England Journal of Medicine*
    www.nejm.org

62. ***NLM Technical Bulletin***
    www.nlm.nih.gov/pubs/techbull/tb.html

63. ***Occupational and Environmental Medicine***
    oem.bmjjournals.com

64. ***Online***
    www.onlineinc.com/onlinemag/index.html

65. **PJB Electronic Publishing**
    www.pjbpubs.com

66. **Scientific American Medicine Online**
    www.sciam.com

67. ***Scrip***
    www.pjbpubs.co.uk/scrip/index.html

68. ***Searcher***
    www.infotoday.com/searcher/default.htm

69. ***The Pink Sheet***
    www.fdcreports.com/pinkout.shtml

ASSOCIATIONS

70. **American Cancer Society**
    www.cancer.org

71. **American College of Physicians-American Society for Internal Medicine (ACP-ASIM)**
    www.acponline.org

72. **American Dental Association (ADA)**
    www.ada.org

73. **American Hospital Association**
    www.aha.org

74. **Association of Academic Health Sciences Library Directors (AAHSL)**
    www.aahsl.org

75. **Association of Independent Information Professionals (AIIP)**
    www.aiip.org

76. **Association of State and Territorial Health Officials (ASTHO)**
    www.astho.org

77. **Medical Library Association (MLA)**
    www.mlanet.org

78. **Pharmaceutical Research and Manufacturers of America (PhRMA)**
    www.phrma.org

79. **Society of Competitive Intelligence Professionals (SCIP)**
www.scip.org

UNITED STATES FEDERAL GOVERNMENT ENTITIES AND RESOURCES

(Note: Some government databases are also available through commercial aggregators, such as Dialog.)

80. **Agency for Healthcare Research and Quality (formerly Agency for Health Care Policy and Research)**
www.ahrq.gov

81. **AGRICOLA—Agricultural Online Access**
www.nal.usda.gov/ag98

82. **AIDSDRUGS; AIDSLINE; AIDSTRIALS**
igm.nlm.nih.gov

83. **CANCERLIT**
cancernet.nci.nih.gov/cancerlit.html

84. **CancerNet**
cancernet.nci.nih.gov

85. **ClinicalTrials.gov**
clinicaltrials.gov

86. **Complementary and Alternative Medicine Citation Index**
nccam.nih.gov/nccam/resources/cam-ci

87. **Environmental Protection Agency (EPA)**
www.epa.gov

88. **FDA Consumer**
www.fda.gov/fdac

89. **Food and Drug Administration (FDA)**
www.fda.gov

90. **GENE-TOX (Genetic Toxicology/Mutagenicity Data Bank)**
sis.nlm.nih.gov/sis1

91. **Grateful Med**
igm.nlm.nih.gov

92. **Hazardous Substances Databank (HSDB)**
sis.nlm.nih.gov/sis1

93. **HealthSTAR**
igm.nlm.nih.gov

94. **IBIDS**
odp.od.nih.gov/ods/databases/ibids.html

95. **Integrated Risk Information System (IRIS)**
sis.nlm.nih.gov/sis1

96. **MEDLINE**
www.nlm.nih.gov/databases/medline.html

97. **MEDLINE*plus***
medlineplus.nlm.nih.gov/medlineplus

98. **National Cancer Institute**
www.nci.nih.gov

99. **National Center for Complementary and Alternative Medicine (NCCAM)**
nccam.nih.gov/nccam

100. **National Center for Health Statistics**
www.cdc.gov/nchs

101. **National Health Interview Survey**
www.cdc.gov/nchs/nhis.htm

102. **National Institutes of Health (NIH)**
www.nih.gov

103. **National Library of Medicine**
www.nlm.nih.gov

104. **NIH Clinical Trials**
clinicaltrials.gov

105. **NIH Consensus Guidelines**
consensus.nih.gov

106. **NIOSHTIC**
www.cdc.gov/niosh/nioshtic.html

107. **NTIS—National Technical Information Service**
www.ntis.gov

108. **Office of Dietary Supplements**
dietary-supplements.info.nih.gov

109. **OMIM—Online Mendelian Inheritance in Man**
www.ncbi.nlm.nih.gov/Omim

110. **Partners in Information Access for Public Health Professionals**
www.nnlm.nlm.nih.gov/partners

111. **PDQ**
cancernet.nci.nih.gov/pdqfull.html

112. **PubMed, PubMed Central**
www.ncbi.nlm.nih.gov/PubMed

113. **RTECS (Registry of Toxic Effects of Chemical Substances)**
www.cdc.gov/niosh/rtecs.html

114. **TOXLINE**
     sis.nlm.nih.gov/sis1

115. **TOXNET**
     sis.nlm.nih.gov/sis1

OTHER GOVERNMENT ENTITIES AND RESOURCES

116. **BadgerLink (Wisconsin Department of Instruction)**
     www.dpi.state.wi.us/dpi/dltcl/badgerlink

117. **EUDRAnet (European Agency for the Evaluation of Medicinal Products)**
     www.eudra.org

118. **Medical Board of California**
     www.medbd.ca.gov/Verifica.htm

119. **Northern Wisconsin Area Health Education Center, Inc. (NAHEC)**
     www.dwave.net/~nahec

120. **RISKLINE (Utah Department of Health)**
     www.health.state.ut.us/cfhs/he/prl/service.html

121. **Therapeutics Products Programme of Health Canada**
     www.hc-sc.gc.ca/hpb-dgps/therapeut

DATABASES

(Note: Some databases are available directly from the producer or via the Web; others are available through commercial aggregators.)

122. **Allied and Complementary Medicine (AMED) (British Library Healthcare Information Service)**
     Available on Dialog, Ovid, and others.
     library.dialog.com/bluesheets/html/bl0164.html

123. **BIOSIS Previews (BIOSIS)**
     www.biosis.org

124. **CAB Abstracts (CAB International)**
     www.cabi.org

125. **Canadian-International Nurse Researcher Database**
     nurseresearcher.com

126. **CenterWatch.com**
     www.centerwatch.com

127. **CINAHL (CINAHL Information Systems)**
www.cinahl.com

128. **Cochrane Collaboration; Cochrane Controlled Trials Register; Cochrane Database of Systematic Reviews**
hiru.mcmaster.ca/cochrane

129. **Cornell University Material Safety Data Sheets**
See Material Safety Data Sheets

130. **Database of Abstracts of Reviews of Effectiveness (DARE) (University of York)**
nhscrd.york.ac.uk

131. **EMBASE (Elsevier Science)**
Available on Dialog, Datastar, Ovid, and others.
www.elsevier.com/inca/publications/store/5/2/3/3/2/8

132. **ERIC (National Library of Education)**
www.accesseric.org

133. **Gale's Health and Wellness Database (The Gale Group)**
Available on Dialog and others.
library.dialog.com/bluesheets/html/bl0149.html

134. **IMSWorld Product Launches (IMSWorld)**
Available on Dialog, Datastar, CAS, and others.
library.dialog.com/bluesheets/html/bl0446.html

135. **IMSWorld R&D Focus (IMSWorld)**
Available on Dialog, Datastar, CAS, and others.
library.dialog.com/bluesheets/html/bl0445.html

136. **Index to Dental Literature**
Included in all versions of MEDLINE.

137. **International Nursing Index (INI; Lippincott Williams & Wilkins)**
Included in all versions of MEDLINE.
www.lww.com/cgi-bin/wwonline.storefront/
808966388/Product/View/0020&2D8124

138. **International Pharmaceutical Abstracts (American Society of Health-System Pharmacists**
Available on Ovid, Dialog, Datastar, and Cambridge Scientific Abstracts.
www.csa2.com/detailsV3/ipa.html

139. **Investext (The Investext Group)**
Available on Dialog, Factiva, and others.
www.investext.com

140. **ISI Citation Indexes; ISI Web of Science**
See SciSearch

141. **MANTIS (Manual Alternative and Natural Therapy) (Healthindex)**
Available on Dialog, DataStar, Ovid, and others.
www.healthindex.com/MANTIS.asp

142. **Material Safety Data Sheets**
msds.pdc.cornell.edu

143. **NAPRALERT**
national.chiropractic.edu/academ/napralert.html

144. **NME Express (New Molecular Entity Express) (Prous)**
Available through Dialog, DataStar, and others.
www.prous.es/product/electron/nme.html

145. **Pharmaprojects (PJB Publications)**
Available through Dialog, Ovid, CAS, and others.
www.pjbpubs.co.uk/pharma

146. **PsycINFO (American Psychological Association); PsycLIT**
www.apa.org/psycinfo

147. **SciSearch (ISI Citation Indexes) (Institute for Scientific Information)**
Available through Dialog, DataStar, STN, Web of Science, and others.
www.isinet.com

148. **Sigma Theta Tau International's Registry of Nursing Research**
www.stti.iupui.edu/rnr

GENERAL SEARCH ENGINES

149. **AltaVista**
www.altavista.com

150. **HotBot**
hotbot.lycos.com

151. **Infoseek (now known as Go.com)**
infoseek.go.com

152. **Lycos**
www.lycos.com

153. **Yahoo!**
www.yahoo.com

DATABASE VENDORS/AGGREGATORS

154. **DataStar**
   products.dialog.com/products/datastarweb/index.html

155. **Dialog**
   www.dialog.com

156. **Dow Jones**
   www.dowjones.com or djinteractive.com

157. **Northern Light**
   www.northernlight.com

158. **Ovid Technologies**
   www.ovid.com

159. **STN**
   stnweb.cas.org

MISCELLANEOUS

160. **Caredata.com**
   www.caredata.com

161. **Cyber Dialogue**
   www.cyberdialogue.com

162. **EBSCO**
   www.ebsco.com/home

163. **eHealthCareWorld Trade Show**
   www.ehealthcareworld.com

164. **EduCause**
   www.educause.edu

165. **"Exploding head syndrome" hoax**
   www.lunaticlounge.com/fringefiles/explode.html

166. **McMaster University**
   www.mcmaster.ca/home.html

167. **Micromedex**
   www.micromedex.com

168. **OCLC (Online Computer Library, Inc.)**
   www.oclc.org

169. **ProQuest**
   www.bellhowell.infolearning.com/proquest

170. **U.S. Pharmacopeia**
www.usp.org

171. **University of Michigan Cancer Center**
www.cancer.med.umich.edu

172. **University of Michigan Document Center**
www.lib.umich.edu/libhome/Documents.center

173. **University of Pennsylvania Biomedical Library**
www.library.upenn.edu/biomed/

ELECTRONIC DISCUSSION LISTS

174. Medical librarians discussion list (MEDLIB-L)
Note: Membership in Medical Library Association not required.
To subscribe, send a message to listserv@listserv.acsu.buffalo.edu.
Leave the subject line blank. In the message type:
SUBSCRIBE MEDLIB-L yourfirstname yourlastname

175. SLA Pharmaceutical Division discussion list (sla-dphm)
Note: Membership in Special Libraries Association required.
See www.sla.org.
To subscribe, send a message to lists@lists.sla.org.
Leave the subject line blank. In the message type:
subscribe sla-dphm yourfirstname yourlastname

CITED LITERATURE, STUDIES, AND BOOKS

176. "Alternative therapies moving toward the mainstream: Doctors are teaching each other alternative medical procedures like acupuncture," CNN, February 23, 1999. Web posted at: 11:16 p.m. EST
www.cnn.com/HEALTH/9902/23/alternative.mds

177. Buyse, Mary Louise, ed. (1990). *Birth Defects Encyclopedia*. Dover, Mass.: Blackwell Science, Inc.

178. "The Core of the Bibliographic Apple: Access to Periodicals for Allied Health Sciences Professionals," presented May 17, 1993, MLA Nursing and Allied Health Sciences Section Program: Supporting the Information Needs of an Allied Health Clientele. Summary published in *NAHRS Newsletter*, 1993 (November) 13(2): 17-21.
www.library.kent.edu/nahrs

179. Dietary Supplement Health and Education Act of 1994.
vm.cfsan.fda.gov/~dms/dietsupp.html

180. Eisenberg study. www.ama-assn.org/sci-pubs/sci-news/ 1998/snr1111.htm#joc80870

181. Gehanno J. F., Paris C., Thirion B., Caillard J. F., "Assessment of Bibliographic Databases Performance in Information Retrieval for Occupational and Environmental Toxicology," *Occupational and Environmental Medicine*, 1998 Aug; 55(8):562-6. www.ncbi.nlm.nih.gov/cgi-bin/Entrez/referer?/htbin-post/ Entrez/query%3fdb=m&form=6&uid=9849544&Dopt=r

182. Hardman, J. G., et al. (1995). *Goodman & Gilman's: The Pharmacological Basis of Therapeutics*, ninth edition. McGraw Hill Ryerson. www.mcgrawhill.ca/medical/g&g.htm

183. Haynes, R. B., Wilczynski, N., McKibbon, K. A., Walker, C. J., Sinclair, J. C., "Developing optimal search strategies for detecting clinically sound studies in MEDLINE." *Journal of the American Medical Informatics Association*, 1994 Nov-Dec; 1(6):447-58. www.amia.org/pubs/jamia/v01n06/447.htm

184. Hill, D. R., "Brandon/Hill selected list of books and journals for the small medical library." *Bulletin of the Medical Library Association*, 1999 Apr., 87(2):145–169. www.allenpress.com/mla/issues/vol87/number2/87-2-145.html

185. McKibbon, Ann (1999). *PDQ: Evidence-Based Principles and Practice*. Hamilton, Ontario: B. C. Decker, Inc. www.bcdecker.com

186. Rugge, Sue and Alfred Glossbrenner. *The Information Broker's Handbook*, 3rd Ed., 1997. New York: McGraw-Hill. Out of print.

187. Sackett, David L., W. Scott Richardson, William Rosenberg, and R. Brian Haynes (2000). *Evidence-Based Medicine: How to Practice and Teach EBM (Evidence-Based Medicine)*, London: Churchill Livingstone. cebm.jr2.ox.ac.uk/docs/bookcontents.html

Appendix B:
Glossary of Terms

1938 Food, Drug and Cosmetic Act. Federal act that included the requirement that new drugs be demonstrated as safe before marketing.

Acrobat format. File format used by Adobe Systems' Acrobat software, permitting documents to be presented exactly as they appear in their original print form. Often referred to as **PDF** (**P**ortable **D**ocument **F**ormat).

AHCPR. Agency for **H**ealth **C**are **P**olicy and **R**esearch, now Agency for Healthcare Research and Quality. Government agency that studies the relationships between medical care, policy, and society.

Alternative medicine. Also known as **complementary medicine**. Treatments and healthcare practices that are not widely taught or used by Western medical professionals.

Armamentarium. The set of implements used by surgeons and physicians, similar to the arsenal of a military officer.

Boolean searching. A logical search process in which keywords are combined using AND, OR, and NOT in order to ensure that the resulting documents contain, or do not contain, the specified terms. For example, *meat AND potatoes* requires that the document contain both terms; *meat OR potatoes* requires that the document contain at least one of those terms and possibly both; *meat NOT potatoes* requires that the document contain the first term but not the second.

BRS. A database vendor purchased by Ovid Technologies in 1994.

CAS Registry Number. Unique registry number given to each chemical by Chemical Abstracts Service. Used for precise chemical searching in many chemical and medical databases.

Case report. A published report on a single patient, usually for the purpose of illustrating an unusual set of symptoms, therapy, or response to therapy.

Clicks & mortar. Retail companies with both a physical and an Internet sales presence, e.g., Barnes & Noble, J. C. Penney.

Complementary medicine. Also known as **alternative medicine**. Treatments and healthcare practices that are not widely taught or used by Western medical professionals.

Diagnosis. The art or act of identifying a disease from its signs and symptoms.

Dialindex. Dialog search system feature that allows researchers to test search terms across several databases simultaneously, in order to determine which databases might contain the information being sought.

Double-blind study. An experimental procedure in which neither the subjects nor the experimenters know the makeup of the test or control groups during the actual course of the experiments.

Etiology. Cause or origin of a disease or medical condition.

Evidence-Based Medicine (EBM). Clinical discipline in which the clinician is aware of the best evidence from clinical and healthcare research, and brings that knowledge into practice at the bedside, in the surgery or clinic, and in the community.

Explode (in database searching). Function used in searching a database, such as MEDLINE, that maintains a thesaurus in outline form. **Explode** permits the searcher to expand a single thesaurus term in order to include all the terms listed under that term. For example, in MEDLINE, *EXPLODE Keratitis* would retrieve results indexed under Acanthamoeba Keratitis, Corneal Ulcer, Keratitis Herpetic, Keratoconjunctivitis.

Health informatics. Information technology applied to improve the communication and management of medical information, as opposed to focusing on the content of that information. Also known as **healthcare informatics**.

HMOs. Health Maintenance Organizations, a system of managed care in which members or their employers pay a set fee or premium each month in return for access to a network of doctors, hospitals, and healthcare services.

Index Medicus. The basis for MEDLINE; a monthly listing of references to current articles from more than 3,200 of the world's biomedical journals.

Internet Syndrome. Clinician name for situations in which consumers believe they know the cure for certain diseases or disorders, based on their reading of medical literature on the Web.

Litigation preparation. Obtaining the documentation one might require for making a claim, including checking résumés, finding articles written by an expert witness, and obtaining relevant statistics, e.g., "20 percent of MRIs are false negatives."

Litigation support. Finding case law or precedent-setting decisions to support a legal position.

Mainstream medicine. Treatments and healthcare practices generally taught and used by Western medical professionals. Sometimes called **traditional**, **conventional**, or **Western medicine**.

Material Safety Data Sheet. A document that provides basic information on a material or chemical product, including properties and potential hazards of the material, how to use it safely, and what to do in case of an emergency.

M.B.A. Master's in Business Administration.

MEDLARS. **MED**ical **L**iterature **A**nalysis and **R**etrieval **S**ystem; the computerized system of databases and databanks offered by the National Library of Medicine.

Megatrends. Popular 1982 book by author John Naisbitt, which characterized America's shift from industrial production to providing services and information.

MeSH. **Me**dical **S**ubject **H**eadings, the National Library of Medicine's controlled vocabulary thesaurus, which forms the indexing structure for MEDLINE.

Meta-analysis. The statistical analysis of the analyses of large numbers of individual studies, for the purpose of integrating the findings.

Metasite. Web site devoted to a single subject, providing links to other sites related to the same subject. Used interchangeably with **subject hub.**

M.L.S. Master's in Library Science.

NIH. National Institutes of Health.

NIH Consensus Guidelines. Independent reports developed by National Institutes of Health Consensus Development Conferences, which are convened to evaluate specific biomedical technologies.

NTIS. National Technical Information Service, the United States Federal government's central source for the sale of scientific, technical, engineering, and related business information produced by or for the U.S. government, and complementary material from international sources.

OneSearch. Dialog search system feature that allows the searcher to run the same search across several databases simultaneously.

Pharmacognosy. The study of the physical, chemical, biochemical, and biological properties of drug substances of natural origin, as well as the search for new drugs from natural sources.

Pharm.D. Doctor of Pharmacy.

Pipeline. Products currently under development with an aim towards commercialization. Generally used with reference to pharmaceuticals or medical devices being developed by manufacturers.

PowerPoint. Microsoft presentation software.

Practice guidelines. Statements that bring together the best external evidence and other information regarding a specific health problem, in order to guide a clinician's decisions with respect to that problem.

PreMEDLINE. The National Library of Medicine's in-process database for MEDLINE, containing basic citation information and abstracts, and available before the citation is indexed with NLM's MeSH heading. Accessed through PubMed.

Prognosis. Expected course of a disease or medical condition, given its current status.

SGML. Standard Generalized Markup Language, an international standard for representing texts in electronic form, independent of device or system.

Subject hub. Web site devoted to a single subject, providing links to others sites that are related to that same subject. Used interchangeably with **metasite**.

Therapy. Treatment of a physical, mental, or behavioral disorder.

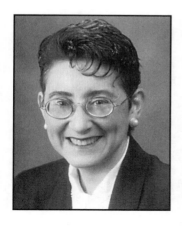

About the Author

Susan M. Detwiler has been working at the conjunction of healthcare, business, and information since 1976. She is a researcher, consultant, and speaker, and a regular contributor to the *Medical and Healthcare Marketplace Guide*, *Medical Industry Information Report*, and *CBSHealthwatch*. Along the way, she has produced the annual *Detwiler's Directory of Health and Medical Resources*, available in hardcopy and various venues online, and has written for numerous information and medical device industry publications.

After receiving an M.B.A. and B.S. in business administration, Susan worked in market research for nine years in the medical device industry, then started The Detwiler Group in 1985. She is a member of the Medical-Surgical Marketing Research Group, of which she is past president, the Association of Independent Information Professionals, the Special Libraries Association, and the Midwest Health Marketers Association.

Susan resides in Fort Wayne, Indiana, with her husband, two children, and a cat. She is connected to the world via fax, phone, modem, and Fort Wayne International Airport. She can be reached at sdetwiler@detwiler.com.

About the Editor

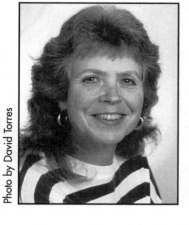

Photo by David Torres

Reva Basch, executive editor of the Super Searchers series, is a writer, editor, and consultant to the online industry. She is the author of the original Super Searcher books, *Secrets of the Super Searchers* and *Secrets of the Super Net Searchers*, as well as *Researching Online For Dummies* and *Electronic Information Delivery: Ensuring Quality and Value*. She writes the "Reva's (W)rap" column for *Online* magazine, has contributed numerous articles and columns to professional journals and the popular press, and has keynoted at conferences in Europe, Scandinavia, Australia, Canada, and the U.S.

A past president of the Association of Independent Information Professionals, she has a Master's in library science from the University of California at Berkeley, and more than 20 years of experience in database and Internet research. Reva was Vice President and Director of Research at Information on Demand and has been president of her own company, Aubergine Information Services, since 1986.

She lives with her husband and three cats on the Northern California coast.

Index

More CyberAge Books
from Information Today, Inc.

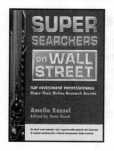

Super Searchers on Wall Street
Top Investment Professionals Share Their Online Research Secrets
Amelia Kassel • Edited by Reva Basch

Through her probing interviews, Amelia Kassel reveals the online secrets of ten leading financial industry research experts. You'll learn how information professionals find and analyze market and industry data, as well as how online information is used by brokerages, stock exchanges, investment banks, and individual investors to make critical investment decisions. The Wall Street Super Searchers direct you to important sites and sources, illuminate the trends that are revolutionizing financial research, and help you use online research as part of a powerful investment strategy. As a reader bonus, a directory of top sites and sources is hyperlinked and periodically updated on the Web.

Softbound • ISBN 0-910965-42-0 • $24.95

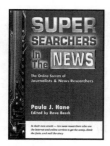

Super Searchers in the News
The Online Secrets of Journalists & News Researchers
Paula J. Hane • Edited by Reva Basch

Professional news researchers are a breed apart. The behind-the-scenes heroes of network newsrooms and daily newspapers, they work under intense deadline pressure to meet the insatiable, ever-changing research needs of reporters, editors, and journalists. Here, for the first time, ten news researchers reveal their strategies for using the Internet and online services to get the scoop, check the facts, and nail the story. If you want to become a more effective online searcher and do fast, accurate research on a wide range of moving-target topics, don't miss *Super Searchers in the News*. As a bonus, a dedicated Web page links you to the most important Net-based information sources—Super Searcher tested and approved!

Softbound • ISBN 0-910965-45-5 • $24.95

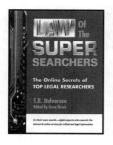

Law of the Super Searchers
The Online Secrets of Top Legal Researchers
T.R. Halvorson • Edited by Reva Basch

In their own words, eight of the world's leading legal researchers explain how they use the Internet and online services to approach, analyze, and carry through a legal research project. In interviewing the experts, practicing attorney and online searcher T.R. Halvorson avoids the typical introductory approach to online research and focuses on topics critical to lawyers and legal research professionals: documenting the search, organizing a strategy, what to consider before logging on, efficient ways to build a search, and much more. *Law of the Super Searchers* offers fundamental strategies for legal researchers who need to take advantage of the wealth of information available online.

Softbound • ISBN 0-910965-34-X • $24.95

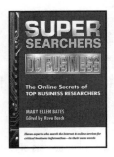

Super Searchers Do Business
The Online Secrets of Top Business Researchers
Mary Ellen Bates • Edited by Reva Basch

Super Searchers Do Business probes the minds of 11 leading researchers who use the Internet and online services to find critical business information. Through her in-depth interviews, Mary Ellen Bates—a business super searcher herself—gets the pros to reveal how they choose online sources, evaluate search results, and tackle the most challenging business research projects. Loaded with expert tips, techniques, and strategies, this is the first title in the exciting new "Super Searchers" series, edited by Reva Basch. If you do business research online, or plan to, let the Super Searchers be your guides.

Softbound• ISBN 0-910965-33-1 • $24.95

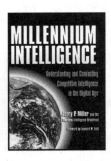

Millennium Intelligence
Understanding & Conducting Competitive Intelligence in the Digital Age
Edited by Jerry P. Miller

With contributions from the world's leading business intelligence practitioners, here is a tremendously informative and practical look at the CI process, how it is changing, and how it can be managed effectively in the Digital Age. Loaded with case studies, tips, and techniques, chapters include What Is Intelligence?; The Skills Needed to Execute Intelligence Effectively; Information Sources Used for Intelligence; The Legal and Ethical Aspects of Intelligence; Small Business Intelligence; and Corporate Security and Intelligence.

Softbound • ISBN 0-910965-28-5 • $29.95

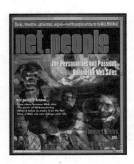

net.people
The Personalities and Passions Behind the Web Sites
Thomas E. Bleier and Eric C. Steinert

With the explosive growth of the Internet, people from all walks of life are bringing their dreams and schemes to life as Web sites. In *net.people*, authors Bleier and Steinert take you up close and personal with the creators of 35 of the world's most intriguing online ventures. For the first time, these entrepreneurs and visionaries share their personal stories and hard-won secrets of Webmastering. You'll learn how each of them launched a home page, increased site traffic, geared up for e-commerce, found financing, dealt with failure and success, built new relationships—and discovered that a Web site had changed their life forever.

Softbound • ISBN 0-910965-37-4 • $19.95